EARTH
ENERGY
MEDITATIONS

EARTH
ENERGY
MEDITATIONS

Awaken Your Root Chakra—
The Foundation of
Well-Being

SUSAN SHUMSKY, DD

WEISER
BOOKS

This edition first published in 2021 by Weiser Books, an imprint of
Red Wheel/Weiser, LLC
With offices at:
65 Parker Street, Suite 7
Newburyport, MA 01950
www.redwheelweiser.com

ISBN: 978-1-57863-703-4

Library of Congress Cataloging-in-Publication Data available upon request.

Cover and text design by Kasandra Cook
Cover image © Shutterstock.com

Typeset in Palatino
Printed in Canada
MAR
10 9 8 7 6 5 4 3 2 1

Disclaimer

Earth Energy Meditations can introduce you to the complex field of meditation, visualization, affirmation, and mantra, but in no way claims to fully teach the techniques described. This book is not an independent guide for self-healing. Susan Shumsky is not a medical doctor and does not diagnose or cure diseases or prescribe treatments. No medical claims are implied about any methods in this book, even if specific "benefits" or "healing" of conditions are mentioned. Readers are advised to consult a medical doctor or psychiatrist before using any methods in this book. Susan Shumsky, her agents, assignees, licensees, and authorized representatives, as well as Divine Revelation, Teaching of Intuitional Metaphysics, and Red Wheel/Weiser, make no claim or obligation and take no legal responsibility for the effectiveness, results, or benefits of reading this book, of using the methods described, or of contacting anyone listed in this book or at *www.divinerevelation.org;* deny all liability for any injuries or damages incurred; and are to be held harmless against any claim, liability, loss, or damage caused by or arising from following any suggestions made in this book, or from contacting anyone mentioned in this book or at *www.divinerevelation.org.*

From the Author

This book is dedicated to those loving, sensitive, open, gentle souls who absorb external vibrations as a sponge absorbs water. This book provides the key to self-authority and unlocks the door to inner strength. Behind that door you will find your true self.

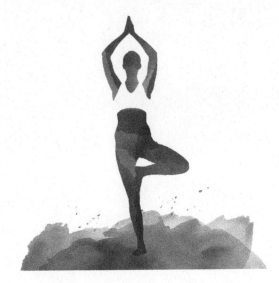

Contents

Introduction

How to Meditate with This Book

Though over 14 percent of American adults say they practice meditation, many do not achieve a deep state of restful alertness. Therefore, they are not getting the anticipated relaxing, healing, spiritually uplifting results. This book can provide an answer. It offers a simple, enjoyable way to meditate—"guided meditation." This easy method can produce practical, positive results for anyone.

WHAT IS "GUIDED MEDITATION"?

Guided meditation is an effortless way to be led step-by-step, moment-by-moment through the process. Just read the words from the page, which guide you into deep meditation and awaken your higher being. Or for even better results, record the words onto your electronic device. Then play back the meditation at a low volume and follow the simple instructions.

Practicing these meditations can infuse your body, mind, and spirit with energy, strength, love, and happiness. You can receive divine inspiration, healing, and wisdom, and develop charisma and magnetic attraction. You can glow with vital well-being. You can stay grounded while awakening your spiritual self.

Guided meditation requires no special abilities, talent, skill, expertise, effort, training, preparation, or practice. There is no need to wrench your body into pretzel positions, sit uncomfortably with a rigid spine, force out thoughts, blank your mind, or strain to concentrate.

In this book you are not asked to "watch your breathing" (or similar ineffectual advice). Instead, you are guided through each meditation in detail, step-by-step. It is best to record the words of each meditation onto your phone, tablet, or computer. Speak softly, slowly, soothingly, and gently. When you come to ellipses (. . .) in the text, that indicates a pause, so record a few moments of silence. Then play back the meditation while sitting comfortably with eyes closed, and your own voice will guide you into meditation. It is that simple!

The book is written in a particular order to help you gain increasing strength and integrity. So it is best to practice these meditations in the order they are written. However, if you wish to explore a particular subject in your meditation practice, you may focus on specific chapters.

WHAT IS "VISUALIZATION"?

This book guides you into meditation as you imagine, with your mind's eye, what is being described. However, believing you cannot "visualize" will not hinder your success. You do not need any special skill to achieve good results. Just follow the directions on the page, step-by-step, which take you progressively deeper into meditation.

Visualization can be difficult when you strain to focus or concentrate on making pictures in your mind's eye. But these guided meditations do not require that. These are simple instructions to follow, which lead you into meditation automatically.

WHAT IS "AFFIRMATION"?

Another method in this book is "affirmation." I call these "spoken meditations." These powerful statements, verbalized audibly, can change your outlook instantly. They remove blockages and clear a pathway for deeper experiences, and effect positive change for yourself and the planet.

Buddha tells us, in the first verse of the first chapter of the Dhammapada (the essential Buddhist scripture):

> *"All that we are is the result of what we have thought: it is founded on our thoughts, it is made up of our thoughts. If a person speaks or acts with an evil thought, pain follows him*

or her, as the wheel follows the foot of the ox that draws the
carriage . . . If a person speaks or acts with a pure thought,
happiness follows him or her, like a shadow that never leaves
him or her."[1]

This verse states that we create our own reality primarily through our thoughts, but also speech and actions. It might be difficult to control the random thoughts streaming through your mind daily. But you can easily control your words and deeds.

For example, if you constantly say, "I am so poor, I am so overweight, I am so unhappy, I am so sick," etc., then I guarantee these results will appear in your life. If, on the other hand, you often say, "I am wealthy, I am the perfect weight, I am happy, I am in perfect health," etc., then these results will manifest.

Master Jesus tells us, "Not that which goeth into the mouth defileth a man; but that which cometh out of the mouth, this defileth a man."[2] To become the conscious captain of your ship of destiny, be mindful of your speech. Consciously speak words and engage in actions that support your goals. Affirmations can help.

Some affirmations in this book declare idealistic outcomes that might seem impossible goals. But nothing is impossible in Spirit. Through every thought, word, and deed, you contribute to not only your personal destiny, but also our planetary destiny. You have more power than you could imagine.

Anyone who has ever achieved greatness has done so despite all odds, despite naysayers, and despite self-sabotaging internal demons. It is just a matter of making a fixed decision to fulfill a goal, then making strides through consistency of purpose and persistence in action. It is about moving forward relentlessly, never wavering, and never giving up.

WHAT IS "MANTRA"?

Usually the term "mantra" refers to words in the Sanskrit language that produce beneficial effects. But mantras are affirmations, and they can be in any language. These potent vibrational sounds can be repeated silently in your mind or chanted audibly. In this book you will practice traditional Sanskrit mantras for specific purposes. They can help you get grounded to Spirit, attain higher states of awareness, and achieve your heart's desires. You can recite them in Sanskrit or English, because translations are provided.

WHAT IS THE GOAL OF MEDITATION?

Meditation is the best way to speed up your spiritual evolution and expand your awareness. After meditating for over fifty years, I believe meditation is the panacea of all ills. It returns you to center, makes you relaxed and content, and heals all kinds of problems. Just by meditating, pains vanish, emotions stabilize, and happiness grows.

The guided meditations in this book are called "earth energy meditations" because they help you become more grounded and attuned to your own nature and the natural world. Practicing them develops your natural gifts of clairvoyance, clairaudience, and clairsentience. As you become more sensitive to subtle experiences, you can travel to wondrous, ecstatic destinations in inner space.

Above all, if you are willing to practice meditation regularly, you can open the doorway to the ultimate goal: infinite consciousness. You can realize who you really are. You can become yourself.

Let us get started with guided meditation practice, now!

Part I

Rooted in Spiritual Security

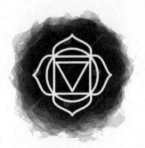

Chapter 1

Are You an Energy Sponge?

A s residents of advanced civilization, obsessed with technology, we live in emotional isolation. Subject to a relentless assault of toxic messages, energies, and brain-numbing activities, we idolize glamour, fame, and money, and we marginalize learning and spirituality. Our constant craving for material things causes the kind of pressure, anxiety, and stress that was unthinkable in previous centuries.

Because of the unbelievable demands we face daily, there is a new pathology: "Highly Sensitive Person (HSP)"—empathic people who absorb energy as a sponge absorbs water. Do you feel drained by the surrounding polluted physical and mental atmosphere? Do energy vampires and toxic relationships suck you dry? Perhaps you feel bodily pain when sensing people's negative emotions. Congestion in crowded situations may overwhelm you. You might feel drained by people all day, until, by evening, all you can do is collapse.

As HSPs or "energy sponges," we have become allergic to poisonous foods, contaminated air, and noxious electromagnetic frequencies. Our sleep is disturbed by geopathic energies and pollution from artificial light. We suffer energy drain symptoms, such as negative emotions, psychosomatic pains, tension, and agitation. We overreact to slights and feel easily hurt and rejected. Unfair, aggravating, annoying situations distress us. We beat ourselves up and compare ourselves with others. We feel embarrassed and compelled to hide our emotions.

Why are we so sensitive? Today we have lost our connection with the earth and any sense of tradition. We have forgotten our roots and pay no respect to the giants on whose shoulders we stand. We feel lonely and in pain. We might try to quell the emptiness by medicating ourselves into oblivion with addictive substances or behaviors. Our lives have been reduced to tiny screens on hand-held devices that induce a perpetual hypnotic trance. Live interaction, camaraderie, and humanity have largely disappeared.

What does this have to do with "earth energies"? In a word— everything. Unless we return to our earth connection, we will be lost. It is time to get grounded in our true nature as a child of Mother Earth, before it is too late. Where to begin our return home? Perhaps by examining our own energy field, we can find an answer.

Chakras (in Sanskrit) are energy centers in your "vital body" that give life to your physical body. *Muladhara,* the "root chakra" at the base of your spine in your tailbone, links you to the earth. When this chakra is closed, muddied, and unhealthy, you experience HSP symptoms of fear, timidity, worry, doubt, anger, frustration, panic, self-loathing, survival mode, defensiveness, and you manifest addictions, narcissism, aggressive behavior, bullying, and entitlement or victimhood.

This book offers potent treatments for these maladies. Powerful, easy-to-use methods of guided meditation, affirmation, visualization, mantra, breathing, and physical movements can reconnect you with primal earth energies. You can reap the benefits of an open, clear, and healthy root chakra, and return to stability, security, and centered well-being. You can enjoy strength of character, integrity, perseverance, persistence, self-acceptance, self-worth, practicality, healthy survival instinct, and prosperity.

SELF-EMPOWERMENT AFFIRMATION

Let us begin with the most powerful energy injection in this book. By affirming self-empowerment in a strong, authoritative voice, with conviction, you can immediately lessen HSP symptoms.

Speak this affirmation audibly whenever you feel weakened, drained, anxious, fearful, overwhelmed, intimidated, or nervous. Say it upon leaving your home, before sleep or meditation, before an interview, audition, or date, before and after meeting a client, and any apprehensive situations. It can center and ground you instantly. I strongly recommend verbalizing this affirmation daily.

I AM in control.
I AM the only authority in my life.
I AM divinely protected by the light of my being.
I close off my aura and body of light
To the lower astral levels of mind
And I open to the spiritual world.
Thank you God, and SO IT IS.

HEALING ENERGY-DRAIN SYMPTOMS

Defeat energy-drain symptoms by giving yourself an instant energy-injection and vitality infusion. Say these potent words audibly whenever you feel drained or out of sorts. This affirmation is calming and soothing, and it brings inner strength.

I call upon my higher self to release, loose, and let go of all
negative thoughts, feelings, and emotions that have caused me
to feel drained of energy. I now release all thoughts and emotions
of oversensitivity, overwhelm, depletion, drain, exhaustion,
pressure, stress, anxiety, apprehension, nervousness, and fear.

These thoughts are now lifted, healed, released, dissolved, and let go into the divine light. And they are gone. They are burnt in the fire of divine love.

I now welcome, embrace, and accept new, powerful, positive thoughts and emotions of integrity, inner strength, invincibility, infinite replenishment, infinite energy infusion, infinite vitality, inspiration, ease, comfort, effortlessness, trust, support, love, and joy. I AM in control. I AM the only authority in my life. I AM divinely protected by the light of my being. Thank you God, and SO IT IS.

DEFEATING ENERGY VAMPIRISM

Some energy vampires might be controlling you through passive-aggressive or guilt-tripping manipulations. Perhaps they are obsessed with you or seek to sabotage you. You do not have to be subject to leeches and parasites that are sucking your energy dry. You can drive a stake through the heart of energy vampirism with these healing words. Speak this affirmation audibly and clearly, with conviction, whenever you feel a psychic vampire is draining your energy:

I call upon Spirit to lovingly cut psychic ties, karmic bonds, and binding ties between myself and all energy vampires that have been draining me. I now cut any and all binding ties between myself and (name or names of energy vampires). These ties are now lovingly cut, cut, cut, cut, cut, cut, cut, cut, cut, cut, cut, cut, cut, cut, lifted, loved, healed, released, dissolved, and let go, in the light of divine love and truth.

I AM in control. I AM the only authority in my life. I AM divinely protected by the light of my being. I AM filled and surrounded with an armor of divine light and divine love. Nothing and no one can diminish the fullness of my being. I AM complete and whole. I AM unassailable. I AM the perfection of being. I AM perfection everywhere now. I AM perfection here now. Thank you God, and SO IT IS.

"ROOTED IN EARTH" VISUALIZATION

This meditative visualization can help you become grounded and rooted in Mother Earth, and more mentally and emotionally stable, physically strong, spiritually lifted, and graceful in movements. Though reading these words can be beneficial, it is best to record them onto your device, such as a computer. Speak softly, slowly, soothingly, and gently. Then play back the recording at a low volume while sitting comfortably with eyes closed. When you come to ellipses (. . .) in the text, pause for a few moments. When an affirmation is part of the meditation, and you see ellipses (. . .), please pause long enough to repeat that part of the affirmation. Here is the meditation:

Please sit comfortably in a chair or a couch and close your eyes. Please keep your eyes closed until I tell you to open them. Now plant your feet firmly on the floor. Imagine your body is like a tree, and the tree trunk is your spinal column. That tree is straight, tall, rigid, immovable, and impenetrable. Now visualize roots of that tree growing downward from the base of your spine, reaching from your spinal column downward and downward, until those roots penetrate the earth below you. The roots continue to spread deep into the earth. Feel yourself rooted deep into the earth's soil. Even if a gale blows fiercely, you remain firmly planted in the earth. The roots continue to grow, penetrating deeper and deeper, giving to your body, mind, and emotions great stability, strength, and solidity.

You now feel a profound connection with Mother Earth. The roots attached to your spine, which have deeply penetrated the earth, are now soaking up Mother Earth's vital, nourishing life energy. This powerful life energy now flows upward through your spine and then spreads all over your body as it enlivens and revitalizes your being on every level: physical, mental, emotional, and spiritual. That life energy is like liquid light, flowing up your spine and then spreading throughout your circulatory system. That light now circulates all over your body, invigorating, energizing, and vitalizing you. That light now becomes brighter and more powerful. Imagine the light is now penetrating and pervading every part and particle of your being as it increases in brightness and intensity. Your body is now filled with brilliant radiant light—the light of life energy. Stay in the silence for a few moments and enjoy the radiant liquid light of life . . . [Record 15 seconds of silence here.]

Now it is time to come out of meditation. Have the intention to return to inner and outer balance. Then pretend to blow out four candles by leaning forward very slightly in your chair and blowing out forcefully through your mouth four times . . . [Record 10 seconds of silence here.]

Then, when you feel ready, open your eyes. If you still feel like keeping your eyes closed, blow out more candles . . . [Record 5 seconds of silence here.] Then open your eyes and repeat the following affirmation audibly:

I AM alert . . . I AM very alert . . . I AM awake . . . I AM very awake . . . I AM inwardly and outwardly balanced . . . I AM in control . . . I AM the only authority in my life . . . I AM divinely protected . . . by the light of my being . . . Thank you God, and SO IT IS.

ROOT CHAKRA CHANT

This chant and visualization can help ground you to earth energies, provide a stable foundation, and improve your centeredness, security, and ease of movement. Your "root" or "base" chakra is at the base of your spine. Activating this chakra enlivens the densest of nature's five elements (earth, water, fire, air, and ether), which are building blocks of all creation. That is the earth element. To learn more about the elements (a.k.a. *tattwas*), please read *The Big Book of Chakras and Chakra Healing.*

Here is how to practice:

Sit in a chair with feet flat on the floor, or sit on the floor or the ground with back support. Imagine your base chakra is firmly planted in the earth, like a tree. Take a few deep breaths. As you inhale, place your attention on the root chakra and tighten the muscles of your anus. As you exhale, relax your pelvic muscles and place attention on your brow chakra at the forehead. (See image on page 162 to find the location of the chakra points.)

Then continue to breathe deeply. On the inhale, place attention on the root chakra and tighten the muscles of your anus. Then as you exhale, relax your pelvic muscles and chant the word LAM, as you continue to place attention on the root chakra while you imagine the sound LAM vibrating in the chakra.

To learn how to pronounce the mantra and chant along, please search the HariomWaley channel on YouTube for "'Lam' Beej Mantra - 'Lam' Seed Mantra," or search the Meditative Mind channel on YouTube for "Magical Chakra Meditation Chants for Root Chakra | Seed Mantra 'LAM.'"

MOTHER EARTH MANTRA

Chant this mantra audibly 108 times to invoke and offer salutations to Mother Earth. This increases your attunement to the earth element, the earth plane, and the nourishment of our beautiful planet Earth, which supports and heals you.

OM Bhu Mataye Namaha

Here is how to pronounce it: OM Bhoo-Mah-tah-yay Namaaha
Here is the translation: OM and salutations to Mother Earth.

MOTHER EARTH MEDITATION

This meditation can help you attune to the earth by communing with nature. It can ground, center, and invigorate you. Practice it outdoors where you can connect with and draw upon earth energies.

Go outdoors and take off your shoes in a place where you will feel comfortable in bare feet, such as a sandy beach, a garden, or on the grass. Stand straight and tall on the earth in your bare feet. Become aware of the feeling of your feet connecting with the earth. Imagine your feet merging into the earth beneath you. Visualize becoming one with the earth as your feet fully connect with the earth.

Then see a channel running from the top of your head, down through the midline of your body, down through the soles of your feet, and then down, down, down, into the heart of the earth. Imagine your bare feet now sprouting roots or cords that are penetrating the earth and running downward farther and farther, down, down to the center of the earth. Visualize that you are exchanging life energy with the earth and that connection is getting stronger and stronger.

Then take a walk in bare feet and imagine that connection with the earth strengthening with every step you take. If there is a tree nearby, sit or stand with your back against the tree. Align your spine against the tree. Then, as you inhale deeply, imagine you are breathing in the life force energy of the tree. As you exhale, feel the exchange of life energy with the tree. Then continue to breathe deeply and visualize the tree and the earth feeding you energy through your spine.

Whenever you wish to reconnect with the earth, you can revisit this experience by visualizing the cord of energy and roots that connect you to the earth.

QUICK SELF-AUTHORITY AFFIRMATIONS

Whenever you notice you are undergoing HSP symptoms, you can speak any or all of these quick affirmations audibly, with power and conviction, to return you to center:

I AM that I AM.
I AM here now.
I AM safe.
I AM secure.
I AM protected.
I AM exactly where
I AM supposed to be.
I AM enough exactly as I AM.
I AM loved.
I forgive myself.
I accept myself.
I love myself.
Thank you God, and SO IT IS.

Chapter 2

Healing Astral Entities

Many spiritual leaders tend to discount the idea of the astral plane and entities that live in that world. They contend their students should focus only on love and light. In a way they are right—that is, if this planet were an ideal heavenly paradise. However, it is unrealistic to imagine that we humans, who live in a negative world where we are dealing with internal and external demons daily, should just ignore the astral plane and pretend it does not exist. Especially if we are HSPs.

I believe if you want to develop spiritually, it is essential to learn about the astral plane and its denizens. In this chapter you will discover what entities are, how to tell when they are present, and how to heal them, using visualization and affirmation methods.

You have undoubtedly heard about NDEs (Near-Death Experiences), where people flatline and undergo a temporary death and then return to life to report what they experienced on the other side. Most report at least one of the following: seeing a divine light of immeasurable glory, seeing a tunnel where deceased loved ones usher them into the light, going into the light, having a life review, meeting a divine being or beings, and choosing to return to earth.

I believe NDEs are real, and they show us what really happens after death. When humans experience death, their souls usually go into the divine light. However, in *Awaken Your Divine Intuition* and in *Divine Revelation,* I deal extensively with the reasons some souls do not enter that divine light after death. I also recommend *The Unquiet Dead* by Edith Fiore.

HSPs are likely to be negatively influenced and feel drained by astral entities. Usually the entities are lost, sad, and confused, because they are stuck and stranded in the astral plane. But some are manipulative and cunning and have a specific agenda. Others are demonic beings that make the astral plane their home. Astral entities will sometimes attach themselves to living humans for a variety of reasons.

"Astral influence" means an entity is nearby and you feel its negative presence. "Astral oppression" is a strong negative energy where the entity is hanging around and influencing you. "Astral possession" means the entity has attached itself to you and is cohabiting your body. Entity possession cannot supplant your soul, but it can crowd you out, change your personality, turn you into an addict, cause a psychotic break, or create mental illness.

How do you know whether an entity is influencing you? Here are possible signposts:

Astral Influence:

- You feel a dense, heavy, negative vibration or get a creepy feeling.

- You feel excessive fatigue, lethargy, or depression.

- You are unusually angry or bad-tempered.

- You do not feel like yourself.

- You feel out of sorts.

Astral Oppression:

- You are abnormally drained and feel something is sucking you dry.

- You undergo a lot of bad luck or misfortunes.

- You often have nightmares.

- You have strong negative emotions and feel out of control.

Astral Possession:

- You have a sudden personality change that is not for the better.

- You get negative telepathic messages, voices, or hallucinations.

- You have a sudden craving for drugs, alcohol, or other addictive behaviors that you never had before.

- You undergo a psychotic breakdown.

SPIRITUAL EXORCISM

This first method for healing astral entities is quite simple. These souls are stuck in the astral plane and need to cross over into the light. So, whenever you sense their presence, simply ask them to go into the light. I recommend speaking audibly the following, or something similar:

Dear beloved soul. You are lost and confused and stuck in the astral plane. But there is no need to be afraid. Look for the divine light, which is filled with warmth and unconditional love. That light is always there. You can simply ask for it to appear. When you see the light, walk toward it and enter it. Do

not fear. Now look for that light. Go into the light, and be at
peace.

HEALING EARTHBOUND SPIRITS

Earthbound spirits are human souls who did not go into the divine light after death. Therefore they are bound to the earthly, material world and have not moved on. Please speak this healing affirmation audibly to help them find their way home:

Dear beloved ones. You are unified with the truth of your being. You are lifted into the divine presence. You are surrounded with divine light and filled with divine love. You are forgiven and healed of all loss, sadness, fear, and pain. You are free from this earthly vibration. You are no longer bound to the material world. You are free to go into the divine light now. You are blessed, forgiven, and released into the love, light, and wholeness of universal Spirit. You are blessed, forgiven, and released into the love, light, and wholeness of universal Spirit. You are blessed, forgiven, and released into the love, light, and wholeness of universal Spirit. You are lifted into divine light. You are lifted into divine light. You are lifted into divine light. Go now to your perfect right place of expression. Go now into the light, in peace and in love.

HEALING DEMONIC SPIRITS

Demonic spirits are astral entities with negative intentions. Their motive is to cause harm through manipulation, control, and fear. They might display poltergeist activity, such as moving furniture; rattling windows; turning lights, radio, or television on or off; or creating chaos. You can heal them by speaking this healing affirmation audibly:

Dear beloved being. I know you live in fear and pain. I realize you feel unloved and alone. I know you are suffering and unhappy. However, there is a way out of the hell you are in. Now it is time to lift yourself out of this deplorable state. You are not cursed. You have a choice to remain in misery, or to change. It is your choice whether to remain in depression, or rise above it. By simply asking for the divine light to appear, you can transform your life now.

You do not need to live in fear. The divine light is always there, and you can call upon it now. Within you is a divine spark, and you can nurture that spark to grow into a great flame. Call upon the divine light now and move toward it. See the light and feel its brilliance. It is the light of Spirit, and it exudes unconditional love. Now is the time to enter the divine light and let go of all misery and suffering. Move into the light now and do not look back. Go now in peace and love.

HEALING FAKER SPIRITS

Faker spirits are frustrated souls that inhabit the astral world. When they walked the earth, they craved name, fame, and recognition, but did not get it. Then after death, they try to become famous by attaching themselves to a psychic medium or channeler. They might ascribe themselves a fake name, such as a religious or Biblical name, in order to impress and deceive humans. These faker spirits then channel their message through the medium by speaking or by writing a book. Healing faker spirits is difficult because there is a symbiotic relationship between the medium and the entity. If the medium is getting financial gain or notoriety, the medium would not want to let the entity move on. However, you can heal a faker spirit by speaking the following affirmation:

*I call upon the divine presence to heal and release this spirit.
Dear one, you are healed and forgiven. You are unified with your
true nature of being. You are filled and surrounded with divine
love and light. You are free from the need to attach yourself to a
human. I now call upon the divine presence to cut any and all
psychic ties, binding ties, and karmic bonds between this faker*

spirit and me. These psychic ties are now lovingly cut, cut, cut, cut, cut, cut, cut, cut, cut, cut, lifted, loved, healed, dissolved, released, and completely let go into divine light and truth.

You are now forgiven of your need to gain name, fame, and fortune. You can now let go of your obsession that has caused you to hide your identity. No longer are you ashamed of being yourself. No longer do you need to be something you are not. I now call upon the divine presence to heal and lift you out of material existence. I call upon the divine presence to help you to discover who you really are and to embrace your inner truth and cosmic identity. You are now lifted in divine love and light. You are now free to go into the divine light. You are now free to express your real nature and to experience the truth of your being. Go now into the divine light. Go now in peace and love. Be at peace, dear one. Be at peace.

Chapter 3

Protecting Your Energy Field

In any spiritual work, divine protection is essential. If you meditate or receive intuitive impressions, it is mandatory to protect yourself from earthbound spirits, demonic entities, energy vampires, and other negative vibrations. I highly recommend affirming and visualizing divine protection and also increasing your inner core spiritual stability. The affirmations and meditations in this chapter can help.

SPHERE OF SACRED PROTECTION

To overcome HSP energy drain and increase inner stability, this meditation can help you visualize a protective sphere around your energy field. Please speak softly, slowly, soothingly, and gently as you record this meditation onto your device and then sit comfortably and play it back at a low volume. When you see ellipses (. . .) while reading and recording the text, please pause for a few seconds.

Please sit comfortably and close your eyes. Keep your eyes closed until I tell you to open them. I now call upon Spirit to surround you in love. Love is the only presence and only power in this universe. Love is within you and all around you. This cosmos is conceived of and perpetuated by love. You are deeply loved by the lover that created you and everything else in this universe. This love now pervades and permeates your being, filling you with warmth, comfort, security, and peace.

Now imagine that the divine light of the almighty creator shines brightly in an infinite sphere above you. That light is beauteous, radiant, and glorious. There is nothing as bright, brilliant, and magnificent as this divine sphere. It is filled with boundless love of inconceivable radiance and splendor. Now picture a ray of this brilliant light shining down from this sphere. It now radiates onto your head and penetrates the top of your skull . . . This pure ray of divine light now streams down through your head and then all the way down your spinal column to the base of your spine . . . Your spine is now lit up with this bright divine light . . .

Now picture this divine light beginning to grow and spread from your energy centers, known as chakras, along the spine. Think of these centers as little suns in your spine that begin to vibrate, radiate, and spread this divine love and light throughout your body. These centers are at the base of your spine, your genital area, your navel, your heart, your throat, and your forehead. They are glowing, vibrating, and growing larger and brighter. As they radiate, they begin to fill your entire body.

Imagine this brilliant light pervading your entire body. But the light does not stop at the edge of your body. It now suffuses and surrounds you. This light becomes a radiant golden sphere that engulfs you and encompasses your entire energy field. You are immersed in this light. It surrounds you with beauty, grace, and glory. You are blessed by this sphere of light, and you are divinely protected . . .

Now it is time to come forth from this meditation. Take a few deep breaths and pretend you are blowing out four candles . . . . [Record 10 seconds of silence here.] Then open your eyes and repeat this affirmation after me:

I AM alert . . . I AM awake . . . I AM in control . . . I AM one with Spirit . . . I AM the only authority in my life . . . I AM divinely protected . . . by the light of my being . . . I AM safe, secure, and protected . . . in this divine sphere of light . . . Thank you God, and SO IT IS.

BUDDHA PROTECTION

This is a visualization to use for divine protection, increased awareness, and well-being. Please record this onto your device in a soft, slow, soothing voice, and then play it back and follow the instructions.

Sit comfortably and close your eyes. Please keep them closed until I tell you to open them. Take a big deep breath of relaxation. Breathe in . . . And out . . . Take a big deep breath of inner peace. Breathe in . . . And out . . . Take a big deep breath of divine light. Breathe in . . . And out . . . Then breathe normally. Peace, peace, be still. Be still and be at peace. Perfect peace, perfect peace, perfect peace. Be still and be at peace.

Now imagine that Spirit is filling your body and aura with divine love . . . Waves of unconditional love are now cascading into and through your entire energy field, pervading it with ecstatic oneness . . . Spirit is now streaming divine light into your aura and filling your entire energy field with beauteous radiant light . . . Spirit is now flooding your aura with currents of divine grace and blessings . . .

Now visualize that your energy field is being blanketed with divine protection. It is now encased in a strong, thick, but resilient covering that brings strength, safety, security, and fortification. Now imagine that you are the Buddha, sitting in meditation cross-legged under the bodhi tree. Visualize that your energy field is now vibrating and pulsating. Your aura is radiating divine energy and emitting the glow of pure love, light, peace, wisdom, and compassion. Spend a few moments in this blissful state . . . [Record 30 seconds of silence here.]

Now it is time to return from this meditation. Take a few deep breaths and pretend that you are blowing out at least four candles . . . [Record 10 seconds of silence here.] Then open your eyes and say this affirmation audibly in a powerful, positive voice:

I AM alert . . . I AM awake . . . I AM in control . . . I AM the only authority in my life . . . I AM divinely protected . . . by the light of my being . . . Thank you God, and SO IT IS.

SECURITY IN THE SELF

Here is an affirmation, to be spoken audibly, which can bring you back to center and help you feel fully integrated in your true self:

I AM that I AM.
I AM the oneness of being.
I AM the perfection of being.
I AM perfection everywhere now.

I AM perfection here now.
I AM whole, complete, and fully integrated.
I live in the center of being.
I dwell in the heart of God.
Thank you God, and SO IT IS.

AFFIRMATION OF DIVINE PROTECTION

James Dillet Freeman, a Unity Church minister, composed this affirmation during World War II to give comfort to soldiers in the trenches. Speak this affirmation audibly, with conviction, whenever you feel the need for divine comfort, safety, and security.

The light of God surrounds me.
The love of God enfolds me.
The power of God protects me.
The presence of God watches over me.
Wherever I AM, God is, and all is well.

MEDITATION FOR SELF-PROTECTION

This meditation can help you experience divine protection. It is best to record this onto your device in a soft, soothing, gentle, quiet voice. Then play back the recording at low volume.

Sit comfortably and close your eyes. Please keep them closed until I tell you to open them. We now know that Spirit is the divine protector. Spirit is our only shelter and only security. Spirit is the loving protector of all its children in the universe. Spirit is wholeness and oneness. Spirit is one and only one. Spirit is one without a second. Spirit is perfection everywhere now. Spirit is perfection here now.

We are now fully merged and one with Spirit, our divine protector and only shelter. We are that center of perfect protection within. There is no separation between ourselves and Spirit. We are where Spirit is. We are now in the loving presence of Spirit's enveloping security and protection. We dwell in the sanctum sanctorum that Spirit is. Spirit's loving presence fills us now with peace, security, wholeness, and oneness. We are safe and secure in Spirit's loving arms. Wherever we are, Spirit is. Wherever Spirit is, we are.

We now therefore claim perfect security and protection, now and always. We live in the sanctuary of the most high. We wear the armor of Spirit. We dwell in the innermost hidden cave in the heart of God. We embrace the holy heart of divine love. Therefore we are protected and filled with the radiance of divine love and peace. We reside under God's umbrella of pure protection, safety, and security. No one and nothing can assail or diminish us. We are whole and complete. We are pure and stainless in our innermost being. We live in integrity.

Love is the only power and the only presence in this universe and in our lives. Love is all we need to be free. We dwell in the heart of divine love. Love is within us and all around us. God's love defines us. We are children of the almighty, born of divine love. God's love is within us and spreads everywhere around us. This love is our armor of protection, safety, and security.

We are now united with the invincible loving presence of Spirit. We are never alone. For Spirit is with us now and always. We are wrapped in the cocoon of God's perfect love. And we emerge as the butterfly—glistening, beauteous, and radiant. From the heart of the most high, we emerge and are set free. We live in the glorious presence of God's love. Free as a butterfly, displaying our true colors boldly, without fear.

We are residents of the holy sanctuary of God's love—divinely protected, divinely inspired, divinely led, divinely filled, and joyously expressing our true nature without fear. We live in the heart of God. We dwell in the house of the Lord. We thank Spirit for this divine protection. We are divine messengers. We are divine philanthropists. And we thank God that this is so now, and SO IT IS.

Now we come forth from this meditation with gratitude in our hearts. Let us pretend to blow out four candles . . . [Record 10 seconds of silence here.] Then we come all the way out to inward and outward balance and open our eyes. Say this affirmation audibly with eyes open:

I AM alert ... I AM very alert ... I AM awake ... I AM very awake
... I AM inwardly and outwardly balanced ... I AM in control ... I
AM the only authority in my life ... I AM divinely protected ... by
the light of my being ... Thank you God, and SO IT IS.

I AM SPIRIT AFFIRMATION

Say the following affirmation audibly, with conviction, to declare your oneness with Spirit. Where there is only one, there can be no other. Nothing and no one can diminish or weaken oneness. It is unassailable and invincible, simply because there is no other.

I AM the love that Spirit is.
I AM the light that Spirit is.
I AM the joy that Spirit is.
I AM the presence that Spirit is.
I AM the good that Spirit is.
I AM the perfection that Spirit is.
I AM the glory that Spirit is.
Thank you God, and SO IT IS.

AARONIC BENEDICTION

This ancient invocation and blessing, adapted from the Bible, Numbers 6:24-26, is very powerful and produces immediate positive results. Here is my version, rewritten in first person. Say it audibly with heartfelt feeling.

> *The Lord bless me, and keep me:*
> *The Lord make his face shine upon me,*
> *And be gracious unto me:*
> *The Lord lift up his countenance upon me,*
> *And give me peace.*

ST. PATRICK'S BREASTPLATE

St. Patrick's Breastplate is a popular invocation for protection, attributed to Ireland's most beloved patron saint. It was written in 433 A.D., before St. Patrick successfully converted the Irish King Lóegaire and his subjects to Christianity.[1] Say the following words audibly in a strong voice, to invoke a divine armor of protection:

> *I arise today, through*
> *The strength of heaven,*
> *The light of the sun,*
> *The radiance of the moon,*
> *The splendor of fire,*
> *The speed of lightning,*
> *The swiftness of wind,*

The depth of the sea,
The stability of the earth,
The firmness of rock.
I arise today, through
God's strength to pilot me,
God's might to uphold me,
God's wisdom to guide me,
God's eye to look before me,
God's ear to hear me,
God's word to speak for me,
God's hand to guard me,
God's shield to protect me,
God's host to save me.
God with me,
God before me,
God behind me,
God in me,
God beneath me,
God above me,
God on my right,
God on my left,
God when I lie down,
God when I sit down,

God when I arise,
God in the heart of every man who thinks of me,
God in the mouth of everyone who speaks of me,
God in every eye that sees me,
God in every ear that hears me.

DEFEATING ENEMIES MANTRA

Here is an affirmation known as the "Chhinnamasta Mantra" from India's Tantric tradition. Chanting this mantra invokes the Goddess Chhinnamasta—a fierce aspect of the Divine Mother who carries her own severed head in her hand. You can use this mantra to overcome people whose intentions toward you are not beneficial. Please learn how to pronounce the mantra by searching the Internet for "Mahavidya Chinnamasta" on the Julie Hill channel on YouTube.

Shreeng Hreeng Kleeng Aing Vajra Vairochinayee Hum Hum
Phat Swaha

HASHKIVEINU JEWISH PRAYER

This is a prayer for protection to be recited at bedtime. Its purpose is to help you sleep in peace and to return to renewed life the following day. Say this audibly with conviction and confidence:

Grant, O God, that we lie down in peace, and raise us up, our Guardian, to life renewed. Spread over us the shelter of Your peace. Guide us with Your good counsel; for Your Name's sake, be our help. Shield and shelter us beneath the shadow of Your wings. Defend us against enemies, illness, war, famine and sorrow. Distance us from wrongdoing. For You, God, watch over us and deliver us. For You, God, are gracious and merciful. Guard our going and coming, to life and to peace evermore.[2]

PSALM OF DAVID: 27

In this powerful psalm from the Hebrew Bible, King David affirms divine protection. Please repeat this audibly as a powerful affirmation of divine protection:

HaShem is my light and my salvation; whom shall I fear?

HaShem is the stronghold of my life; of whom shall I be afraid?

When evildoers come upon me to eat up my flesh, even mine adversaries and my foes, they stumble and fall.

Though a host should encamp against me, my heart shall not fear;

Though war should rise up against me, even then will I be confident.

PSALM OF DAVID: 121

I have adapted a first-person version of another powerful psalm from the Bible. Repeat this audibly, with confidence, to affirm divine protection:

I will lift up mine eyes unto the mountains: from whence shall my help come?

My help cometh from HaShem, who made heaven and earth.

He will not suffer my foot to be moved; He that keepeth me will not slumber.

Behold, He that keepeth Israel doth neither slumber nor sleep.

HaShem is my keeper; HaShem is my shade upon my right hand.

The sun shall not smite me by day, nor the moon by night.

HaShem shall keep me from all evil; He shall keep my soul.

HaShem shall guard my going out and my coming in, from this time forth and for ever.

PSALM OF DAVID: 91

I have adapted a version in first person of another powerful psalm. You can repeat this audibly as a powerful affirmation of divine protection:

O, I who dwell in the hiding place of the Most High, and abide in the shadow of the Almighty;

I will say of HaShem, who is my refuge and my fortress, my God, in whom I trust,

That He will deliver me from the snare of the fowler, and from the devastating pestilence.

He will cover me with His pinions, and under His wings shall I take refuge; His truth is a shield and a buckler.

I shall not be afraid of the terror by night, nor of the arrow that flies by day;

Nor of the pestilence that walks in darkness, nor of the destruction that destroys at noonday.

A thousand may fall at my side, and ten thousand at my right hand; it shall not come nigh me.

Only with my eyes shall I behold, and see the recompense of the wicked.

For I have made HaShem, who is my refuge, even the Most High, my habitation.

There shall no evil befall me, neither shall any plague come nigh my tent.

For He will give His angels charge over me, to keep me in all my ways.

They shall bear me upon their hands, lest I dash my foot against a stone.

I shall tread upon the lion and asp; the young lion and the serpent shall I trample under my feet.

PROPHET MUHAMMAD'S AFFIRMATION FOR PROTECTION

This affirmation for protection comes from the founder of the Islamic religion, the prophet Muhammad. To invoke God's power and strength, speak it audibly, with conviction:[3]

O God, you are my Lord. There is none worthy of worship except You.

I rely upon You, and You are the Great Lord of the Throne.

Whatever God wills happens, and whatever He does not will does not happen.

There is no power or strength except by God.

I know that God is able to do anything, and that God knows all.

O God I seek refuge in You from the evil in myself and every creature that You have given power over us.

Verily my Lord is on the straight path.

KWAN YIN INVOCATION

Kwan Yin (a.k.a. Avalokiteshvara) is the Buddhist deity of mercy, compassion, and love. In chapter 25 of the *Lotus Sutra*, the Ten Great Deliverance (Salvations) and Protections of Avalokiteshvara are revealed. To call upon Kwan Yin for protection, speak these affirmations audibly, with conviction:[4]

If anyone wishes to harm me by pushing me into the great pit of fire, I invoke the power of Bodhisattva Avalokiteshvara; the inferno pit will be transformed into a water pond. —Lotus Sutra 25: 2.3

If I am drifting in a great ocean and facing imminent danger with dragons, fishes, and other demons, I invoke the power of Bodhisattva Avalokiteshvara; the waves will be unable to swallow me. —Lotus Sutra 25: 2.4

If I am at the summit of Mount Sumeru, and someone pushes me off the edge, I invoke the power of Bodhisattva Avalokiteshvara; I will be suspended in midair like the sun in the sky. —Lotus Sutra 25: 2.5

If I am suffering from the punishment of government, and my life is about to end by execution, I invoke the power of Bodhisattva Avalokiteshvara; the sword will be splintered into pieces. —Lotus Sutra 25: 2.8

If I am being locked in a prison and my hands and feet are being bound by chains and fetters, I invoke the power of Bodhisattva Avalokiteshvara; I will be released and freed. —Lotus Sutra 25: 2.9

If anyone wishes to harm me by curses or poisonous herbs, I invoke the power of Bodhisattva Avalokiteshvara; the effects will be bounced back to the originator. —Lotus Sutra 25: 2.10

If I face harm from vicious rakshasas, poisonous dragons, or various demons, I invoke the power of Bodhisattva Avalokiteshvara; no one will dare to harm me. —Lotus Sutra 25: 2.11

If I am surrounded by evil beasts with sharp fangs and fearful claws, I invoke the power of Bodhisattva Avalokiteshvara; they will quickly flee and scamper away in all directions. —Lotus Sutra 25: 2.12

If I have disputes before the court, or am fearful in the midst of war, I invoke the power of Bodhisattva Avalokiteshvara; all enemies full of resentment will retreat. —Lotus Sutra 25: 2.21

If I wish to give birth to a son, I worship by giving offerings to Bodhisattva Avalokiteshvara, who will bestow me a son blessed with good fortune, virtue, and wisdom. If I wish to have a daughter, I will have a beautiful and adorable daughter blessed with accumulated benevolent roots. —Lotus Sutra 25: 1.11

Part II

Rooted in Spiritual Discernment

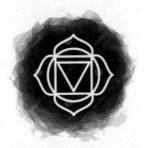

Chapter 4

Developing Inner Wisdom

When trying to make wise decisions, being highly sensitive can cause confusion. There are so many overwhelming energies in today's mad world. How can you know which road to take? Your brain might feel like a jumbled jungle, bombarded by mixed messages from seemingly infinite external and internal sources. Being out of touch with earth energies can pull you in many directions and produce turmoil.

In this chapter, you will learn methods to receive inner guidance, make wise choices with confidence, and elevate your decision-making process. You can become an instrument of the divine and be led by Spirit daily. Interestingly, being an HSP might be an advantage. Sensitive people can readily open to Spirit and receive messages, counsel, inspiration, and inner guidance from the "still small voice" of inner wisdom.

GETTING PRACTICAL GUIDANCE

This meditation can help you listen to the inner voice and receive practical guidance for everyday life. It takes practice and dedication to develop your intuition and discern when it is clear. But this meditation can open the gateway to the flow of inner wisdom. It is based upon one brilliant idea: "Ask, and it shall be given you" (Matthew 7:7).

Please record these words slowly, softly, and gently onto your device. Remember to record plenty of silent time when you see ellipses (. . .). Then play back the recording at a low volume and follow the instructions. Right before listening to this recording, please drink a glass of water, speak audibly the Self-Empowerment Affirmation on page 6, and use the three energy-infusing exercises on pages 65 to 71 of this book.

Please sit in a comfortable position with back support. Close your eyes and keep them closed until I tell you to open them. Let's take a big deep breath of divine love. Breathe in . . . And out . . . Let's take a big deep breath of divine light. Breathe in . . . And out . . . And a big deep breath of inner peace. Breathe in . . . And out . . . Then breathe normally. Relax, release, and be at peace. Peace, peace, be at peace. Be still and be at peace.

We now know and recognize that there is one power in one presence at work in the universe and in our lives, the divine presence.

That divine presence is the source of inner wisdom, truth, and inner guidance. It is the repository of knowledge. It is the wise counselor. It is the wayshower on our pathway. It is our divine guide. We are now one with, attuned to, merged with, and fully aligned with the divine presence. There is no separation between ourselves and Spirit. Therefore we are the divine counselor, the wayshower, the divine guide, the wise sage. We now therefore know and claim the perfect meditation for developing intuition right here and now. We ask for all this or better. We now accept in consciousness all that I have spoken or better. And we thank God that this is so now, and SO IT IS.

Let us take a deep breath to go deeper. We now call upon all the divine beings of light to assist us in this meditation. We call forth the Holy Spirit, the spirit of truth and wholeness, to shine the light of truth upon this session. We call forth all the divine beings of light that come in the name of God to assist us in this meditation. We ask the Holy Spirit to clear the pathway so that we may receive clear inner guidance. We call forth the angels and archangels, prophets, and deities to lift our vibration and bring us to higher awareness. We ask that we be led deep within, to the center of being. We know that Spirit is with us and within us, feeding us love, light, power, and energy.

We call forth the grace of God to shower upon us peace, strength, and blessings. We are now lifted to a higher vibration.

We now feel waves of grace coursing into our being, filling us with elevated awareness. The loving presence of Spirit fills and surrounds us now with wave upon wave of divine love. We are touched by the holy presence of Spirit. We are lifted into the ecstatic presence of the Most High. We are filled with the glory of God. We now ask Spirit to lift our vibration even higher. We are floating on waves of ecstasy in an ocean of bliss. We immerse ourselves in divine love and we feel completely at home. Let us enjoy these waves of bliss for some moments in silence . . . [Record 15 seconds of silence here.]

Let us now call upon the Holy Spirit to answer a question that is on our mind. The question is this: "What is my highest and best next step to take on my pathway?" Now take a big, deep breath and ask this question within your own heart: "What is my highest and best next step to take on my pathway?" . . . Then take in a big deep breath . . . And let it go . . . And another deep breath. Breathe in . . . And let go . . . and a third deep breath. Breathe in . . . And let it go . . . Now do what I call "the do-nothing program." That means do nothing, nothing, and less than nothing. Have a neutral, receptive attitude—willing and open to receive. Take another big deep breath. Breathe in . . . And out . . . Then breathe normally. Now allow yourself to be calm and still as you receive the answer to your question . . . Do not seek for the answer. Just let go. Allow the answer to come to you. You might receive it as a vision in your mind's eye, a thought that pops into your mind, or a gut feeling. Just let the answer come to you now . . . [Record one minute of silence here.]

After you have received the answer to your question, give gratitude to God. We will now come forth from this meditation by taking some deep vigorous breaths and pretend to blow out at least four candles. Let us do that now. Vigorously blow out four candles and intend to come all the way out to inward and outward balance . . . [Record 10 seconds of silence here.] Then open your eyes . . . With eyes wide open, let us now repeat audibly the following affirmation:

I AM alert . . . I AM awake . . . I AM very alert . . . I AM very awake . . . I AM in control . . . I AM the only authority in my life . . . I AM divinely protected . . . by the light of my being . . . Thank you God, and SO IT IS.

MAKING WISE CHOICES

Your life is a series of choices, from what you eat for breakfast to what time you go to bed. Every new moment is a chance to make a better choice than you did in the last moment. By reading *Awaken Your Divine Intuition, Miracle Prayer,* and *Divine Revelation,* you can learn how to discover your life purpose, how to discern your best path, how to tell when your intuition is real, and how to make the wisest choices by following clear inner guidance.

This affirmation can help you develop discernment and make the best choices. Speak it audibly with conviction and confidence:

I now see, know, and recognize that my life is a series of choices. Every new moment is a chance to make a better choice than I did in the last moment. Each moment is a chance to make a better life. Every choice I make has consequences that affect my life and the lives of my family, friends, society, and all of humanity. Once I make a choice, I cannot unmake it. Therefore, I call upon my higher self, the source of inner wisdom, to guide me in making the wisest choices in each and every moment.

I AM no longer bound by societal conventions, beliefs, norms, structures, and expectations. I now make choices based on my true heart's desires and true life-purpose and pathway. I look to Spirit rather than to the opinions of others. I search my own heart to discover the wisest path to follow. I now allow my higher self to be my guide. I let go and let Spirit be my best decision maker. I now make a commitment that from this moment, my life is led by my true heart's desires. I allow my divine purpose to unfold with grace and blessedness. I AM at peace, knowing that my higher self is my guide.

GETTING INNER GUIDANCE SIGNALS

How do you know which path to follow? Do you take the red pill or the blue pill? Why is it easy for some people to make the best decisions on a dime, while others waver in doubt and indecision? The truth is people often make choices that are out of alignment with their heart's desires or inner truth. This meditation provides a method to help you make the tough decisions you often face. During the meditation, you will ask Spirit to give you inner "yes" and "no" signals to help you make wise choices with peaceful confidence. I also recommend reading *Divine Revelation*, which includes an entire chapter about how to word and ask questions.

Please record these words slowly, softly, and gently onto your device. Record plenty of silent time when you see ellipses (. . .). Then play back the recording at low volume and follow the instructions. Right before listening to this recording, please drink a glass of water, speak audibly the Self-Empowerment Affirmation on page 6, and use the three energy-infusing exercises on pages 65 to 71 of this book.

Sit comfortably and close your eyes. Please keep your eyes closed until I tell you to open them. We now call upon the Holy Spirit to help you learn how to make decisions with peaceful confidence. During this meditation, we ask the Holy Spirit to give you a "yes" and a "no" signal that you can use to help you make wise choices.

We now know that Spirit is the divine decision maker. Spirit makes no mistakes. Spirit is our divine guide that leads us on our pathway. We now ask Spirit to guide us, to help us discern with great confidence so that we can make the best and wisest choices.

We now call upon the Holy Spirit to take you deep into meditation. Breathe in . . . And let go . . . Take another deep breath of inner peace. Breathe in . . . And out . . . Now take a big deep breath of relaxation. Breathe in . . . And let go . . . Then breathe normally. Deeper, deeper, deeper into the wells of Spirit, into the silence of being. Let go, let go, let go, let go, let go, let go, let God. Peace, peace, peace still. Be still, and be at peace. Allow your body and mind to settle down to inner peace and relaxation. Center your self in inner peace. Let your body and mind relax. Take another deep breath. Breathe in . . . And breathe out . . . Once again, breathe in . . . and breathe out . . . Then breathe normally. You are in a state of deep relaxation and peace. Settle down even more to a state of wholeness and oneness . . . Let your heart be at peace. Allow yourself to enter a state of perfection and unbounded awareness . . .

You are now settled, content, and deeply relaxed. You are in a state of transcendental awareness. Completely relaxed, completely at peace, totally content. Now we call upon the Holy Spirit to give you a "yes" signal. This "yes" signal will now come to you as a vision, a feeling, a sound, a smell, a taste, or an involuntary movement. Take a big deep breath now. And let go. Now do the do-nothing program. Do nothing, nothing, and less than nothing.

Within your heart, say these words now: "Spirit, please feed me a 'yes' signal" . . . Then take a big deep breath and settle down to deep relaxation. Breathe in . . . And out . . . Then breathe normally. Do the do-nothing program, and be receptive to Spirit to receive your "yes" signal. Allow yourself to receive the signal. You will see, hear, taste, smell, or feel something, or get an involuntary movement, something that indicates a "yes" . . . [Record 30 seconds of silence here.]

After you have received the "yes" signal, then say these words now: "Spirit, please feed me a 'no' signal" . . . Then take a big deep breath and settle down once again to inner peace. Breathe in . . . And out . . . Then breathe normally. Now do the do-nothing program, and be receptive to Spirit to allow the "no" signal to come to you . . . [Record 30 seconds of silence here.]

Now it is time to check the signals you have received. Now ask Spirit within your heart, "If the 'yes' signal is what I am thinking it is, please feed it to me now, strong, loud, and clear" . . . Then take a big deep breath and let go. Do the do-nothing program and be receptive. Allow the "yes" signal to come to you . . . [Record 30 seconds of silence here.]

After you receive the "yes" signal clearly, then ask Spirit within your heart, "If the 'no' signal is what I am thinking it is, please feed it to me now, strong, loud, and clear" . . . Then take a big deep breath and let go. Do the do-nothing program and be receptive. Allow the "no" signal to come to you . . . [Record 30 seconds of silence here.]

Once you have checked these inner signals, it is now time to come out of meditation. With gratitude in your heart, now intend to come out of the meditation to inner and outer balance. Now take at least four vigorous breaths and pretend you are blowing out four candles. Do that now. [Record 10 seconds of silence here.] Then open your eyes . . . Then say this affirmation audibly with eyes wide open:

I AM alert . . . I AM very alert . . . I AM awake . . . I AM very awake . . . I AM inwardly and outwardly balanced . . . I AM in control . . . I AM the only authority in my life . . . I AM divinely protected . . . by the light of my being . . . Thank you God, and SO IT IS.

After you have identified clear "yes" and "no" signals, it is wise to practice using them. Before you attempt to get answers to questions, please use these guidelines:

- First drink a glass of water, speak audibly the Self-Empowerment Affirmation on page 6, and use the three energy-infusing exercises on pages 65 to 71 of this book.

- Never ask fortune-telling, predictive questions about the future.

- Ask only one question at a time.

- Ask for highest wisdom and divine guidance rather than should's, should-not's, have-to's, will I, will he, will she, will they, or will this happen.

- Begin "yes" and "no" questions with the following phrase: "Is it highest wisdom for me to _____?"

For more information about using these and other signals, and developing your divine connection safely and effectively, please read my books *Awaken Your Divine Intuition* and *Divine Revelation*.

Chapter 5

Releasing What Does Not Serve You

How can you handle difficult negative emotions, seemingly immovable blocks, and stuck energy? Much of the trials and trauma people endure are related to the root chakra, where the most gripping survival issues get trapped. Although tough challenges might be devastating, there is no need to park your mind in that state for even one minute. In this chapter, you will practice meditations, affirmations, and exercises that can lighten suffering and eliminate what holds you back from realizing the truth.

HEALING TRAUMA

When you hang on to traumatic memories, negative energy gets lodged in your emotional body. This also adversely affects your physical body, possibly resulting in a serious disease. In order to release trauma, this meditation can help. Record these words onto your device in a soft, gentle, slow voice. Then play back the recording at a low volume, and follow the instructions.

Please sit comfortably and close your eyes. Please keep your eyes closed until I tell you to open them. Let us take a big deep breath of relaxation. Breathe in . . . And out . . . Take a big deep breath of inner peace. Breathe in . . . And out . . . Take a big deep breath of divine love. Breathe in . . . And out . . . Then breathe normally. Now relax, relax, release, and be at peace. Peace, peace, be still. Be still, and be at peace. Let us take a big deep breath to go deeper. Breathe in . . . And out . . . And another deep breath to settle down even more. Breathe in . . . And out . . . Then breathe normally.

As you settle down to inner peace, you may notice your attention being drawn inward, into a place within the body that needs attention. You may feel some bodily sensation—a feeling of discomfort, pain, or unease. As you sit comfortably, simply allow your attention to be drawn into that place or places within the body that are drawing your attention. Take another deep breath to go deeper. Breathe in . . . And out . . . Then breathe normally.

Now settle down even deeper into meditation. Allow your attention to rest on the place or places in the body that are drawing your attention . . . Do not try to make the sensations disappear. Do not try to manipulate the sensations. Just notice that they are sensations

. . . [Record 10 seconds of silence here.] In case you feel pain, rather than resisting the pain, just dive into the pain . . . [Record 5 seconds of silence here.] Think of the pain not as pain, but simply as sensation. As you place your attention on that sensation, it will tend to dissipate . . . [Record 10 seconds of silence here.]

Spend a few more moments now quietly feeling the sensation or sensations within your body . . . [Record 20 seconds of silence here.] By placing your attention on these sensations, you are automatically healing the trauma lodged in that part of your body. Allow your breath to dislodge any further energy in the body that no longer serves you. Breathe in . . . And out . . . Then breathe normally. Again place attention on the sensations until they disappear . . . [Record 10 seconds of silence here.] When all the sensations are gone, and your body is comfortable and at peace, just spend a few moments in that inner sanctum sanctorum, your own higher self . . . [Record 30 seconds of silence here.]

When you are ready to come forth from the meditation, just intend to come forth to inward and outward balance as you pretend to blow out four candles and then come all the way back to inner and outer balance . . . [Record 10 seconds of silence here.] With eyes wide open, please say the following affirmation audibly:

I AM alert . . . I AM very alert . . . I AM awake . . . I AM very awake . . . I AM in control . . . I AM the only authority in my life . . . I AM divinely protected . . . by the light of my being . . . Thank you God, and SO IT IS.

UNBLOCKING THE GRANTHI

Three *granthi* (mental/emotional knots) are situated in three energy centers in your subtle body. That is where negative energy, trauma, habits, beliefs, blockages, and destructive feelings get stuck and held. These granthi can cause illness, addictions, pain, or anxiety. In order for *kundalini* (spiritual life energy) to rise up through *sushumna nadi* (the central energy channel in your subtle body), she must break through these knots.

1. Brahma granthi (knot related to physical body) is centered at root chakra and extends to pelvic chakra. Blockages and attachments in this granthi relate to bodily issues, health, genetics, physical vitality, sexuality, procreation, deep desires, and survival instincts.

2. Vishnu granthi (knot related to emotions) is located in heart chakra and includes navel chakra. Blockages, emotions, beliefs, and trauma about love relations, loss, and grief reside in this granthi. So do power struggles, attachments, and repulsions in personal, familial, business, and other relationships.

3. Shiva granthi (related to mind) is situated at brow chakra and extends to throat chakra. Issues with communication, decision-making, mind, speech, intuition, and creative activities reside in

this granthi. So are attachments to psychic powers and arrogance about supernormal abilities.

One way to break through the granthi is to practice *bandhas* (muscular locks). Please see page 151 to learn how. Another way is to practice the following breathing exercise, which you may record on your device and then play back to guide your practice:

Place your attention on the root chakra at the base of the spine. Take a big deep breath through your nose with mouth closed. Inhale while you imagine drawing that breath down, down, down the spine, to the root chakra. Visualize the breath is all concentrated at the base of your spine, as you draw up the muscles of your anus and genitals and squeeze those muscles. Hold your breath at that spot for a few moments . . . [Record 5 seconds of silence here.] Then let go of the breath and also let go of the anus and genital muscles and completely relax. Repeat this process a few times, as you notice that the kundalini energy begins to rise up your spine . . . [Record one minute of silence here.]

Then place your attention on your heart chakra at the center of your chest. Take a big deep breath through your nose with mouth closed. Inhale while you imagine drawing that breath down to the heart center in your chest. Visualize that your breath is all concentrated at the heart and that your rib cage is expanding and your abdomen is tightening. Imagine the deity of your choice is glowing there in your chest as you hold your breath at that spot for a few moments . . . [Record 5 seconds of silence here.] Then let go of the breath and also let go of the ribcage and abdomen and completely relax. Repeat this process a few times, as you notice your heart expanding . . . [Record one minute of silence here.]

Then place your attention on your brow chakra in the middle of your forehead. Take a big deep breath through your nose with mouth closed. Inhale while you imagine drawing that breath up to your forehead. Imagine your breath is all concentrated there in your forehead. See your third eye opening, and light flooding your forehead. Hold your breath at that spot for a few moments . . . [Record 5 seconds of silence here.] Then let go of the breath and completely relax. Repeat this process a few times, as you notice your third eye opening, inner vision awakening, and awareness expanding . . . [Record one minute of silence here.]

Then, when you are ready, with gratitude in your heart, come forth from this exercise and repeat audibly, with eyes wide open:

I AM awake . . . I AM alert . . . I AM inwardly and outwardly balanced . . . I AM in control of my mind at all times . . . Thank you God, and SO IT IS.

CLEARING WASTE

When you cling to worn-out possessions, worn-out ideas, and worn-out relationships that no longer serve you, you limit your spiritual growth. Say this affirmation audibly in a strong, convincing voice in order to remove such clutter from your life.

*I now let go of all worn-out beliefs, habits, ideas, and patterns that
no longer serve me.*
I now let go of all worn-out possessions that no longer serve me.
I now let go of all worn-out relationships that no longer serve me.
I now remove all old clutter from my life on every level:
Physically, mentally, emotionally, and spiritually.
*I no longer need to hold on to old ideas that do not enhance my
spiritual growth.*
*I no longer need to hold on to possessions that have been
possessing me.*
I no longer need to hold on to people that are not enriching my life.
I now let go and invite Spirit into my life.
I now let go of useless ideas, things, and people,
And I make way for Spirit to enter my life.
I now invite and welcome Spirit into my life.
Please fill me with deep peace, abiding love, and brilliant light.
Thank you God, and SO IT IS.

CUTTING BINDING TIES

In order to enjoy positive, powerful, loving relationships, it is wise to cut binding karmic ties daily with all co-workers at your job and loved ones at home. Cutting these negative ties keeps true love bonds healthy and strong. Also, it is wise to cut binding ties with people and things you no longer want to associate with.

To cut these ties, say the following affirmation audibly in a strong, powerful voice. In the blank space, please name one specific person, place, thing, organization, situation, circumstance, memory, or addiction that is unduly influencing you. When using the affirmation, name only one thing at a time. Do not try to cut ties with an entire shopping list. You can learn more about these ties in my book *The Power of Auras*.

I now call upon Spirit to cut binding ties and karmic bonds between myself and _____. These binding ties are now lovingly cut, cut, cut, cut, cut, cut, cut, cut, cut, cut, cut, cut, cut, loved, healed, lifted, dissolved, released, and let go into the light of divine truth. I AM in control. I AM the only authority in my life. I AM divinely protected by the light of my being. Thank you God, and SO IT IS.

EXERCISES FOR AN IMMEDIATE ENERGY BOOST

Are you an energy sponge? Do you feel drained, diminished, or defeated by people you encounter? By practicing highly effective, dynamic, potent, vitality-infusing methods, you can give yourself an energy injection. These simple exercises produce spectacular, immediate results. They can lift your mood, vitality, clarity, and energy instantly. They can clear your energy field and make you centered, balanced, and grounded. They can attune you to earth energies and to your higher self.

These simple yet profound exercises are grounded on Chinese medicine. Anyone can do them. These methods exercise both your body and your brain. They are easy to practice and can be done standing or seated, even at your desk or on a plane.

Before doing these simple movements, drink pure water at room temperature until you feel fully hydrated. By drinking water, your brain and neurons wake up, and you immediately feel more energized.

Infinity Flow

First drink water. Then get a small slip of paper and write an X on it. Hold that paper in your right hand so you can see the X. Sit or stand with your right arm fully extended, directly in front of you. Stare intently at the X, keeping your head still, as your extended right arm and hand traces an imaginary infinity sign in the air, starting from the center of that imaginary figure. Staring at the X the entire time, do not move your head, but move your eyes, so your eyes, arm, and hand are all moving in the infinity pattern.

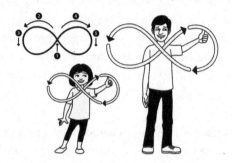

Using your straight right arm, trace up through the middle of the imaginary infinity sign, around one side and down, then up through the middle again, around the other side and down. Repeat that for about 30 seconds. Then place the paper with the X in your left hand and stare at it. Trace the infinity figure again with your straight left arm and hand for about 30 seconds. Then hold the paper with both hands together and trace the figure for another 30 seconds.

Neuro-Linguistic Programming, also known as NLP, tells us that eye movements access different parts of your brain. Tracking an infinity sign with your eyes creates coherence between the brain's left and right hemispheres, and integrates brain functioning. Crossing the body's midline with your arms creates bilateral integration, which improves core stability.

Sit-Down Sit-Ups

I call the next exercise "Sit-Down Sit-Ups" because you will make similar movements as when you practice sit-ups on a floor mat. But this exercise is done standing or sitting.

Drink water if you have not yet done so. Then begin the exercise by lifting your left thigh and briefly touching your left knee with your right elbow. Then lift your right thigh and briefly touch your right knee with your left elbow. Continue alternating like this for about three minutes. As you practice this movement, keep your head still, but look around the room in all fields of vision. At the same time, hum a little tune.

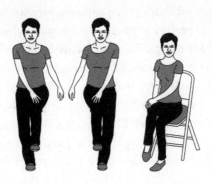

You may practice an easier variation, as seen in the previous image, by lifting your left thigh slightly and then briefly touching it with your right hand. Then lift your right thigh slightly and briefly touch your right thigh with your left hand. Continue to alternate for three minutes. This can be performed either standing or sitting. As you practice this movement, keep your head still, but look around the room in all fields of vision. At the same time, hum a little tune.

This powerful movement improves balance and structural integration. It balances nerve activation across your brain and lights up both brain hemispheres simultaneously. It increases your confidence and reduces anxiety and overwhelm about appearing in public, doing a lecture, being interviewed, or other stressful situations.

Sit-Down Eagle Pose

The Eagle Pose is a difficult yoga posture to practice, but this modified exercise is easy to practice yet produces many of its benefits, plus a few more. The "Sit-Down Eagle Pose" is practiced either seated or standing.

Drink water if you have not yet done so. Then cross your ankles by placing one ankle over the other. Next extend your two arms straight in front of you, with the backs of your hands facing each other (not your palms). Then lift up your right arm a bit and move it to the left. Next, lower your right arm so the palms of your hands face each other. Then interlace your fingers. Keep your fingers interlaced and hands intertwined while relaxing your arms. Let your inter-twined hands descend to your lap, if you are seated, or to your lower abdomen, if you are standing.

You can remain in that position to access your root chakra, or, keeping your fingers interlaced, you can curl your interlaced hands up into a position where your clasped hands are situated right in front of your heart chakra.

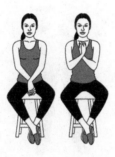

Next close your eyes and take deep breaths, breathing through your nose, with your mouth closed. As you inhale, place your tongue on the roof of your mouth. As you exhale, relax your tongue. Continue to inhale with tongue on the roof of the mouth, and exhale as you relax the tongue. Every time you exhale, imagine you are letting go of stress. Let go more and more with every breath. Continue to meditate like this for about five minutes.

Then open your eyes. Uncross your ankles and uncurl your hands and fingers. Then place the palms of your hands facing each other with just your fingertips touching. In other words, place the fingertips of your left hand on the corresponding fingertips of your right hand, in a steeple position, for about 15 seconds.

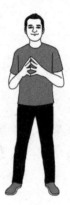

This practice centers, balances, and grounds you. It reduces anger and stress and brings calm, reduces mental chatter, improves focus, and lessens hypersensitivity.

After you have completed these exercises, please speak the following affirmation audibly, with strength and conviction:

I AM in control.
I AM the only authority in my life.
I AM protected, safe, secure, and at peace.

Breathwork for a Change

This exercise increases energy, especially when you feel tired or drained. It helps you release negative energy lodged in your physical and mental body:

Lie on your back on an exercise mat or a bed, completely relaxed. Lightly rest your hands over your solar plexus, just above your navel. Breathe deeply, steadily and rhythmically for a few minutes. Then imagine that as you breathe in, you draw in vital life energy from the universal supply. See this life energy absorbed by your lungs and stored in your solar plexus.

Then as you breathe out, imagine all negative energy is being expelled from your body into the earth below. Imbibe positive, vitalizing energy as you inhale, and release stuck, negative, limiting energies as you exhale. Continue this practice for five to ten minutes.

Chapter 6

Practicing Safe Spirituality

When some people begin to explore spirituality through books, the internet, television, or live events, they become wowed by the promise of psychic phenomena, ancient artifacts, or archeological marvels. It is easy to get enamored with such fascinating arcane mysteries. However, there are hidden dangers in the magical thinking that can sometimes result from such exploration. This chapter can help you avoid the pitfalls of psychic delusion and spiritual materialism.

PERILS OF GLAMOUR

If a psychic or guru seems to display magical properties, your logical mental faculties might turn off, and your irrational emotions could take over. The intrigue, glamour, and mesmerizing effect of charismatic spiritual leaders and occult phenomena could deceive you. It is wise to maintain some semblance of reason when dealing with unknown mysteries. In other words, do not be so open-minded that your brains fall out of your head!

Here is an affirmation to make you more self-reliant and less dependent on gurus or psychics who might not have your highest welfare in mind. Please speak this audibly with conviction in a powerful voice:

I AM in control. I AM one with Spirit. I AM one with my own higher self. I AM safe, protected, secure, and at peace. I call upon Spirit to guide me on my spiritual path. I ask Spirit to show me the truth about seemingly impressive phenomena. I call upon Holy Spirit to fill and surround me with a beautiful bubble of divine protective light. I know this light protects me from spiritual delusion and psychic deception. I AM filled with the light of Spirit. I AM no longer dependent on anyone to guide me. I AM now guided by my own higher self. I AM free from reliance on others. I now depend on my own inner wisdom. I do not need gurus, psychics, readers, or organizations to direct me. I now count on the "still small voice" within to advise me.

I AM the only authority in my life. I AM self-reliant. I now cut psychic ties and karmic bonds between myself and anyone or anything that seeks to control me or take advantage of me. These psychic ties are now lovingly cut, cut, cut, cut, cut, cut, cut, cut, cut, cut, cut, lifted, loved, healed, dissolved, released, and let go into the light of divine truth. I now close off my aura and body of light to anyone or anything that has controlled me. My higher self is my inner counselor. It advises me with highest wisdom. I AM contented, fulfilled, integrated, whole, and complete. Thank you God, and SO IT IS.

FINDING SPIRITUAL SIMPLICITY

Genuine spirituality is not complicated, glamorous, alluring, seductive, or sensational. However, it is blissful. Your true higher self is an experience of simple contentment, which is its true nature. This meditation can help you feel it. Please record these words onto your device in a soft, slow, soothing voice and then play them back.

Please sit comfortably and close your eyes. Keep your eyes closed until I tell you to open them. Let us take a big deep breath of divine love. Breathe in . . . And out . . . Take a big deep breath of divine light. Breathe in . . . And out . . . And a big deep breath of relaxation. Breathe in . . . And out . . . Then breathe normally. We now ask Spirit to come forth and guide us into our true nature, which is inner peace and contentment.

Peace, peace, be still. Be still and be at peace. Perfect peace, perfect peace, perfect peace. Be still, and be at peace. Let us take a big deep breath to go deeper. Breathe in . . . And out . . . Take a big deep breath of inner peace. Breathe in ... And out ... And a big deep breath of wholeness and oneness. Breathe in ... And out ... Then breathe normally. We ask Spirit to take you deeper, deeper, deeper, into the wells of Spirit, into the silence of being. Breathe in ... And out ... Then breathe normally.

Allow your body to settle down to deep relaxation. Completely leg go and relax as you go deep, deep within, into the center of being. Let every part of your body become completely rested and relaxed. Relax your forehead ... your eyes ... your eyebrows ... the space between your eyebrows ... your temples ... your cheeks ... your jaw ... your neck ... your shoulders ... your arms ... your hands ... your fingers ... Relax your chest ... your stomach ... your pelvis ... your buttocks ... your thighs ... your legs ... your knees ... your ankles ... your feet ... your toes ... Relax your forehead ... your eyes ... your eyebrows ... the space between your eyebrows ... Relax your entire body now ...

Peace, peace, be still. Be still and be at peace. Perfect peace, perfect peace, perfect peace. Be still, and be at peace. Take a big deep breath to go deeper. Breathe in ... And out ... Then breathe normally.

Allow your mind to settle down to inner peace ... Your mind now relaxes to inner contentment and perfect peace ... Release, loose, and let go of your mind. Just accept whatever thoughts are coming and going without trying to stop or still or control them. Just let go, let go, let go, let go, let go, let go, let God. Now go even deeper, deeper, deeper, into the silence of being. Breathe in . . . And out . . . Now relax even more deeply. Breathe in . . . And out . . . Then breathe normally.

Now we ask Spirit to fill you with perfect peace. The waves of divine peace are now wafting over you, pervading your being with deep relaxation, serenity, and contentment. You are now filled and surrounded with divine peace, love, contentment, and relaxation. You are now in a deep state of silence and profound relaxation. Let go, let go, let go, let go, let go, let go, let God. Enjoy this state of great contentment for a few moments . . . [Record 15 seconds of silence here.]

When you are ready to come out of meditation, give gratitude in your heart and then pretend you are vigorously blowing out at least four candles . . . [Record 10 seconds of silence here.] Then return to inward and outward balance and open your eyes. Say this affirmation audibly with eyes open, with conviction:

> *I AM alert . . . I AM very alert . . . I AM awake . . . I AM very awake . . . I AM in control . . . I AM the only authority in my life . . . I AM divinely protected . . . by the light of my being . . . Thank you God, and SO IT IS.*

CHOOSING THE BEST MENTOR

How do you know which spiritual teacher *(guru)* to choose or which path to follow? With myriad choices available, and with countless conflicting messages barraging you, this can be confusing. To help you make this pivotal decision, an ancient scripture of India, *The Guru Gita,* can help.

In order to magnetically draw your best teacher into your life, please speak audibly a few verses from this scripture regularly, with confidence and conviction. Almighty forces of nature are eager to help you realize your higher self. When you ask for a mentor with your sincere heart, in faith, these inscrutable forces will bring you and your guru together in a cosmic, serendipitous meeting.[1]

> *The Guru is Brahma, the Guru is Vishnu, the Guru is the Lord Shiva; the Guru is the Supreme Brahman (pure consciousness) himself. I bow to the Guru.*
>
> *I bow to the Guru by whom the eye blinded by the darkness of ignorance has been opened with the salve of knowledge.*
>
> *I bow to the Guru who reveals the true nature of the absolute, which is infinite and indivisible, and which pervades all creation, both moving and nonmoving.*
>
> *I bow to the Guru who reveals the true nature of the soul, which dwells in all creation, both moving and nonmoving.*
>
> *I bow to the Guru who imparts the meaning of that which shows that all the three worlds, consisting of both moving and stationary creatures, are pervaded by pure consciousness (Brahman).*

I bow to the Guru by whose words, even in half a moment or a half or quarter thereof, the firm realization of the higher self is attained.

The letter 'gu' stands for darkness, the letter 'ru' stands for its removal. The Guru is so called because he removes the darkness (of ignorance).

I bow to the Guru, mounted on the power of knowledge and adorned with the garland of reality, who confers prosperity as well as liberation.

I bow to the Guru who, by the power of the fire of knowledge, burns the bondage of karma accumulated over innumerable lives.

I bow to the Guru who shows the way of liberation for those who have got caught in the forest of samsara (the cycle of death and rebirth) and are bewildered by delusion.

All living beings have been bitten by the snake of ignorance. The Lord in the form of knowledge (Guru) is the only physician for them. I bow to the Guru.

The form of the Guru is the object of meditation, the feet of the guru are the object of worship, the words of the Guru are the mantra, and the grace of the Guru is the means of liberation.

Part III

Rooted in Spiritual Integration

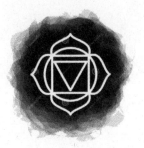

Chapter 7

Accepting Who You Are

A muddy root chakra can bind you to toxic emotions and the miseries of material life. It can keep you chained to ignorance. When you let go of illusion and realize who you really are, you can rise above the false self. This chapter will help you accept who you really are—your true divine self, and eliminate what has kept you bound to your ego.

"I AM" CHANT

The mantra *So Hum* means "I AM." It is an expression of completeness. This mantra can facilitate opening your root chakra, getting grounded in your higher self, developing self-love, realizing who you really are, and accepting that you are enough, exactly as you are right now.

You can use the mantra *So Hum* either by chanting it audibly or repeating it silently. Chanting mantras audibly can unblock and clear your throat chakra, resulting in self-confidence, creative expression, and free-flowing communication. Repeating mantras mentally should not be hammering the words with clear pronunciation. Instead it should be a faint idea—a vibration rather than clear words. When those words fade away, just gently return to them. The fading away of the mantra is more important than remembering to repeat it again.

ACCEPTING EMOTIONS

Many spiritual paths and organizations instruct seekers to refrain from expressing emotions. According to traditions of the Far East, enlightened people are expected to act detached and dispassionate. However, that is a misunderstanding of what enlightenment really is.

The reality is, after you attain spiritual liberation, you will still feel emotions. However, they will no longer overshadow you, because you will not identify yourself with, or as, those emotions. Instead you will remain centered in your higher self while experiencing and expressing emotions.

Here is a meditation to help you accept emotions and not block them. Please read this meditation onto your device in a soft, slow, comforting voice, and then play it back when you are ready to practice it.

Please sit comfortably and close your eyes. Keep your eyes closed until I tell you to open them . . . Peace, peace, be at peace. Be still and be at peace. Let us take a big deep breath of inner peace. Breathe in . . . And out . . . Take a big deep breath of relaxation. Breathe in . . . And breathe out . . . Take a big deep breath of divine love. Breathe in . . . And out . . . Then breathe normally.

We now know that Spirit is the one healing presence and healing power at work in the universe and in our lives. Spirit is freedom of self-expression. Spirit encompasses our whole being, including body, mind, emotions, intellect, ego, and higher self. Spirit encompasses all human experiences, including happiness, sadness, love, hate, contentment, frustration, joy, grief, comfort, and pain. There is nothing missing in Spirit. The realm of emotions is part of it.

We are now merged with, one with, unified with, and the same as Spirit. There is no separation between Spirit and us. Therefore all human emotions and experiences are within us. We now therefore know and claim that you accept your emotions, you nurture your emotional body, and you allow the free flow of emotions in your life.

You now release from your mind all thoughts that have blocked your free flow of emotions. You now let go of all beliefs that spiritual people are not emotional, that they must remain emotionless, that they should not express emotions, and that emotions are a sign of weakness. These false ideas are now lifted, loved, healed, released, dissolved, and let go into the light of divine love. And they are gone. You now welcome new, beautiful, creative thoughts that emotions are spiritual and reflect your higher self, that spiritual people are emotional and it is healthy to express emotions, that being vulnerable and expressing emotions is a sign of strength, not weakness.

Now please take a moment to remember a time when you felt something deeply but you did not express it to a loved one, and you now regret it . . . Now take a few moments to remember that time and relive how it felt to repress that emotion . . . [Record 30 seconds of silence here.] Now go back to that moment in time and play a different movie in your mind's eye. Visualize yourself expressing that heartfelt emotion to that person in a loving and tactful way. Then play the rest of the movie in your inner eye and see how this changed your relationship and changed the outcome of that situation . . . [Record 30 seconds of silence here.]

You now know and accept in consciousness how expression of emotions can have powerful positive effects in your relationships and in your own well-being. So please declare this affirmation audibly in a strong voice, with conviction. Please repeat after me:

I now know and accept . . . that I AM a divine being of light . . . My higher self is a witness . . . to the entire picture show called life . . . My higher self lives . . . in contentment, peace, love, and

serenity . . . At the same time . . . my mental emotional body . . .
continues to function as always . . . All the emotions of human
life . . . are alive and well in my emotional body . . . I no longer
repress, block, or stifle my emotions . . . I allow them to show and
to flow . . . Because I no longer stuff my emotions . . . my body,
mind, and spirit . . . are positive, healthy, strong . . . powerful,
centered, balanced . . . peaceful, serene, and whole . . . Thank you
God, and SO IT IS.

Now come forth from this meditation, with gratitude and love
in your heart. Take four deep vigorous breaths and blow out at least
four candles . . . [Record 10 seconds of silence here.] Then open your
eyes and say the following affirmation audibly:

I AM alert . . . I AM awake . . . I AM inwardly and outwardly
balanced . . . I AM divinely protected . . . by the light of my being
. . . Thank you God, and SO IT IS.

RELEASING YOUR FALSE SELF

Human beings generally identify themselves with the false self, a.k.a.
the ego—limited and bound by ignorance. When I say "ego," I am
not referring to "egotism" or being "egotistical." I am referring to
how you define yourself, i.e., who or what you imagine yourself to

be. For who-you-think-you-are is not who-you-really-are. To begin your journey of discovering your higher self, please speak this affirmation audibly, in a strong voice, with conviction:

I AM not this body. I AM not this name. I AM not the house I live in. I AM not this profession or job. I AM not this history. I AM not the happenings in this life. I AM not these situations and circumstances. I AM not this bank account. I AM not these relationships. I AM not this mother and father. I AM not this spouse. I AM not these children. I AM not any of these loved ones. I AM not this city, state, province, or country. I AM not this political affiliation. I AM not the planet Earth. I AM not the galaxy.

I AM not this mind. I AM not these emotions. I AM not this intellect. I AM not this ego. I AM not this subconscious mind. I am not this aura. I AM not what I refer to as "I." I AM not these senses of seeing, hearing, feeling, tasting, or smelling. I AM not the objects of perception. I AM not what I experience in this world. I AM not these desires. I AM not these goals. I AM not the joy and sorrow I experience. I AM not this birth. I AM not this death. I AM not anything that I can imagine.

I AM what cannot be imagined. I AM the unfathomable. I AM what has never been born and what has never died. I AM the

imperishable. I AM the eternal. I AM the never-ending. I AM
the unlimited, boundless, infinite pure awareness. I AM without
name and form. I AM beyond the material world. I AM the
unmanifest absolute. I AM pure consciousness.

ADI MANTRA

The Adi Mantra creates a meditative link between yourself as a finite, physical, human being, and your higher self as infinite consciousness. By chanting this mantra, you begin to dissolve the human ego and allow universal consciousness to flow through your being. The Adi Mantra can help you open and receive your own subtle inner wisdom and to listen to and trust your inner guidance. Here is the mantra, and you can learn how to pronounce it by searching the Canal Dany Matos YouTube channel for "Adi Mantra (Ong Namo Guru Dev Namo)."

Ong Namo Guru Dev Namo

Here is a translation:

We call upon our highest consciousness to receive, and we call upon our inner divine teacher to guide us.

Chapter 8

Overcoming Shortcomings

You have the power to let go of shortcomings that hold you back from fulfilling your dreams. Many of these negative emotions are lodged in your root chakra, which is the center of survival issues. This chapter can help you become more self-empowered and successful by releasing fears, doubts, timidity, and addictions.

BREAKING THROUGH OBSTACLES

The Hindu deity Ganesha is the beloved elephant-headed trickster that can you help you remove obstacles. This mantra can clear your path when you feel stuck, creatively blocked, or challenged, or you need a different perspective. Chant it audibly when embracing a new mindset, starting a new relationship, beginning a venture, embarking on a journey, taking a plane flight, stalled in traffic, and other challenging situations. To learn how to pronounce the mantra correctly, please search the YouTube channel sainath459 for the video "Ganesh Maha Mantra – Om Gam Ganapataye Namaha."

Om Gam Ganapataye Namaha

Translation:

Salutations to Ganesha, the remover of obstacles, we call your name!

GIVING UP GUILT

Guilt can be paralyzing. It can prevent your moving forward, changing your life, and fulfilling your heart's desires. When guilt makes you feel unworthy and undeserving, it is nearly impossible to reach your goals. But when you feel deserving, you attain your aspirations effortlessly. This meditation can help you heal guilt and shame.

Please read these words onto your device in a soft, slow, soothing voice. Then play back the recording at a low volume. Near the end of this meditation, I have included a Ho'oponopono chant, which is effective for clearing guilt and shame.

Please sit comfortably and close your eyes. Keep your eyes closed until I tell you to open them. Let us take a big deep breath of divine unconditional love. Breathe in . . . And out . . . Let us take a big deep breath of relaxation. Breathe in . . . And out . . . Then breathe normally. Let us open to the presence of divine Spirit. We are held in the arms of divine love. We dwell in the house of the Lord. Let us give up and give over to Spirit. We place our lives in the hands of God.

Now take a few moments to think about past actions for which you feel guilty or ashamed. Imagine yourself in those situations for a few moments now . . . [Record 10 seconds of silence here.] Do not resist looking at these scenarios, and continue to visualize the circumstances under which you have made choices you now regret . . . [Record one minute of silence.]

Now notice that, with the information and level of consciousness you had at the time, it would have been difficult to make different decisions in these cases. Let us now see, know, and accept that whatever you have done in this life or in any past life, in every situation and circumstance you have encountered, you have done the very best you could do, given your level of awareness at that time. Even though you made choices that you now regret, at that time those choices were limited, and your consciousness was also limited. You did what you did, and there is no way to change that, except in your mind.

So at this time, please repeat the following affirmation audibly, with firm conviction and in a powerful voice:

I now completely forgive myself . . . for all my past wrongdoings . . . I know now that I have always . . . done the very best I could do . . . in every situation . . . according to my level . . . of consciousness at the time . . . So I now let go . . . of all regret, guilt, shame, and self-hatred . . . If I could change the past, I would . . . However, I can change the future . . . and I now choose to act . . . in accordance with natural law . . . and the laws of my own higher nature . . .

I now say to myself . . . And to all beings to whom I have done wrong . . . I AM sorry . . . Please forgive me . . . I love you . . . Thank you . . . I AM sorry . . . Please forgive me . . . I love you . . . Thank you . . . I AM sorry . . . Please forgive me . . . I love you . . . Thank you . . . I AM sorry . . . Please forgive me . . . I love you . . . Thank you . . . I AM sorry . . . Please forgive me . . . I love you . . . Thank you . . . I AM sorry . . . Please forgive me . . . I love you . . . Thank you . . . I AM sorry . . . Please forgive me . . . I love you . . . Thank you . . . I AM sorry . . . Please forgive me . . . I love you . . . Thank you . . . I AM sorry . . . Please forgive me . . . I love you . . . Thank you . . . I AM sorry . . . Please forgive me . . . I love you . . . Thank you . . . I

AM sorry . . . Please forgive me . . . I love you . . . Thank you
. . . I AM sorry . . . Please forgive me . . . I love you . . . Thank
you . . . I AM sorry . . . Please forgive me . . . I love you . . .
Thank you . . . I AM sorry . . . Please forgive me . . . I love you
. . . Thank you . . . I AM sorry . . . Please forgive me . . . I love
you . . . Thank you . . . I AM worthy. I AM loved . . . I now
choose to be . . . the best me I can be . . . I now like myself. I love
myself . . . I forgive myself, and I accept myself . . .

Now, with gratitude in your heart, it is time to come forth from
this meditation. Please now take at least four deep, vigorous breaths
and pretend you are blowing out at least four candles . . . [Record 10
seconds of silence here.] Then open your eyes and please repeat this
affirmation:

I AM alert . . . I AM very alert . . . I AM awake . . . I AM very
awake . . . I AM in control . . . I AM the only authority in my
life . . . I AM divinely protected . . . by the light of my being . . .
Thank you God, and SO IT IS.

FEAR CAN DISAPPEAR

Fear is an overpowering emotion that can stop you in your tracks.
Many fears seem irrational, but they are often the result of past life

traumas. For example, if you were a pilot shot down in a fighter plane, you might be terrified of plane flights. If you were branded a witch and burnt at the stake, you may be afraid to reveal your psychic abilities. If you were pushed off a cliff, you might be scared of heights. This meditation can help you heal fears by accessing past life traumas. Please read the words onto your device in a soft, slow, soothing voice. Then play back the recording at a low volume:

Please sit comfortably now and close your eyes. Keep your eyes closed until I tell you to open them. Let us take a big deep breath of divine love. Breathe in . . . And breathe out . . . Let us take a big deep breath of inner peace. Breathe in . . . And out . . . Let us take a big deep breath of relaxation. Breathe in . . . Breathe out . . . Then breathe normally.

Now think about a fear that has been disturbing you. Think about the last time you were in that fearful situation. Remember everything you can about that time and place. Put yourself in that scenario and experience it as vividly as possible. Engage all of your senses. Where are you? . . . What time of day is it? . . . What are you seeing? . . . What are you hearing? . . . What is the weather? . . . What does it feel like? . . . What does it smell like? . . .

Think about how afraid you are. Imagine that being in this situation can cause you great peril. As you put yourself there, think how much this situation terrifies you. Connect with that feeling of fear, and increase the intensity of that feeling. Imagine how scared you are, and double the feeling of fear . . . Then double that fear again . . . Continue to increase the fear until you feel the maximum you possibly can . . . [Record 10 seconds of silence here.] Now remember the first time you ever had this fear in a past life . . . [Record 30 seconds of silence here.]

Now look around you. Where are you? . . . Look down at your clothing . . . Are you male or female? . . . What are you wearing? . . . What time of day is it? . . . What are you seeing? . . . What are you hearing? . . . What is the weather? . . . What does it feel like? . . . What does it smell like? . . . Now ask Spirit to play a little movie in your inner eye where you experience what happened in this past life situation. Take some time to see, hear, and feel what is happening in this past life . . . [Record one minute of silence here.]

Once you have remembered vividly what took place in this past life, now repeat the following affirmation audibly in a clear voice, with conviction:

I AM in control . . . I AM the only authority in my life . . . I AM divinely protected . . . by the light of my being . . . I now see, know and accept . . . that this past life memory . . . is simply a memory . . . I no longer need to fear . . . that this situation will occur again . . . I now let go of all fear . . . And I embrace divine love . . . Where there is divine love . . . fear cannot exist . . .

They cannot occupy the same space . . . I now allow myself to be
loved . . . by the source of love in this universe . . . I now allow
divine love . . . to fill and surround me . . . I let go and let Spirit .
. . fill my heart with love . . . I now allow Spirit . . . to heal me of
all fear . . . I now feel loved, secure . . . protected, and safe . . . in
the arms of divine love . . .

It is now time to come forth from this meditation. Give gratitude to God for this healing. Take four deep vigorous breaths and pretend you are blowing out four candles . . . [Record 10 seconds of silence here.] Then open your eyes and repeat the following affirmation:

I AM alert . . . I AM very alert . . . I AM awake . . . I AM very
awake . . . I AM inwardly and outwardly balanced . . . I AM in
control. I AM the only authority in my life . . . I AM divinely
protected . . . by the light of my being . . . Thank you God, and
SO IT IS.

OVERCOMING ADDICTION

The overpowering craving for addictive substances and activities has an underlying cause. That cause is usually extreme HSP, a.k.a. hypersensitivity. It can manifest as an attack on the senses of perpetual noise from every quarter, of absorbing painful negative emotions and vibrations of others, and of unmanageable emotions. People who cannot cope with reality or with the agony they feel might turn to addictive substances to become comfortably numb.

This meditation can help overcome addictions, whether tobacco, alcohol, drugs, sex, work, shopping, social media, binge-television, or other activities you might bury yourself in to avoid feelings. Please read the words onto your device in a soft, slow, soothing voice. Then play back the recording at a low volume.

Please sit comfortably and close your eyes. Keep your eyes closed until I tell you to open them. Let us take a big deep breath of divine love. Breathe in . . . Breathe out . . . Let us take a big deep breath of inner peace. Breathe in . . . And out . . . Let us take a big deep breath of relaxation. Breathe in . . . Breathe out . . . Then breathe normally.

We now know and recognize that there is one healing power and one healing presence at work in the universe and in our lives, God the good, omnipotent. God is the consummate healer. God is wholeness and oneness. God is perfection everywhere now. God is perfection here now. God is our divine guide, the lighthouse of our life. God is the wayshower on our pathway. God is unblemished, untainted, and pure. God is the source of joy and happiness.

We are one with that divine source. We are the healing presence and healing power that God is. We are God/Goddess incarnate in human form and human flesh. We are ourselves the divine guide, the wayshower, the lighthouse of our life. We are unblemished, untainted, and pure. We are the source of joy and happiness within. We live in the heart of God. We dwell in the house of the Lord. We are unified with, aligned with, and merged with God. God is with us and within us, now and always. We are perfection everywhere now. We are perfection here now.

We now therefore know and claim that you are free from addiction now. Whatever is the cause behind the cause behind the cause of any seeming appearance of addiction in your life—that is now lifted from your mind and heart now, and it is gone.

The need to numb yourself with addiction is now eliminated from your heart. All thoughts, feelings, and emotions that no longer serve are now released from your mind. You now release, loose, lift, and let go of hypersensitivity to toxic internal and external influences that have caused you take refuge in addictive substances and activities that dull your perception. We now call upon Spirit to eliminate all feelings of hypersensitivity, restlessness, physical pain, emotional pain, guilt, remorse, unworthiness, blame, anger, regret, craving, and addiction. These feelings are now healed, lifted, loved, dissolved, released, and let go. They are burnt to ashes in the fire of divine love. And they are gone.

You now welcome and accept into your mind, heart, and soul complete freedom from addiction. You are now filled with powerful, positive, creative thoughts and emotions of inner strength, invincibility, divine security, divine protection, peace, calm, comfort, ease, forgiveness, self-love, self-confidence, self-worth, love, acceptance, contentment, joy, and happiness.

You are now free from addiction and free to be yourself. No longer does addiction rule your life. You are now held in the arms of God and comforted in that loving, divine presence. You no longer have the need to hide and stuff emotions. You allow yourself to live in your physical body and to experience all the feelings that human beings share.

We now call upon Spirit to fill your heart with divine love and to reveal to you your true divine calling, purpose, and heart's desire. We call upon Spirit to show that to you now. Now take a big deep breath. Breathe in . . . And out . . . Then breathe normally. Now take a few moments to see, hear, or feel what Spirit is now showing you . . . [Record 30 seconds of silence here.]

Your life is no longer obsessed with addiction. You are now focused on accomplishing your divine life purpose and passion. You now walk the path of Spirit, and you live in the heart of God's love. Open now to receive waves of divine love, as Spirit blesses you with perfect love and peace . . . Open to receive divine light, which is now streaming into your being . . . Feel the blessings of divine grace flowing into your being . . . You are blessed and beloved of God . . . You are filled with the light of divine love. You are surrounded with divine grace. You are content, and you are at peace . . .

Now, imagine that Spirit is saying to you these words to you: "You are in my heart. You are in my soul. Let me be your strength today, the one who is always with you."

Now, with gratitude in your heart, it is time to come forth from this meditation. Please take at least four deep, vigorous breaths and pretend that you are blowing out at least four candles . . . [Record 10 seconds of silence here.] Then open your eyes . . . With eyes open, please repeat this affirmation:

I AM alert . . . I AM very alert . . . I AM awake . . . I AM very awake . . . I AM in control . . . I AM the only authority in my life . . . I AM divinely protected . . . by the light of my being . . . Thank you God, and SO IT IS.

Chapter 9

Embracing Health and Wealth

By utilizing the methods in this chapter, you can become more integrated in mind, body, and spirit. Practice these meditations, visualizations, affirmations, and exercises to increase well-being and prosperity.

INCREASING PRIMAL ENERGY

In Taoist philosophy, the essence of vital life energy is called jing. This vitality can be lost through ejaculation, menstruation, childbearing, stress, toxic food, fluorinated water, addictive substances, profligate lifestyle, and aging. However, vitality can be restored through herbal preparations or meditative practices.

This simple yet profound exercise instantly increases the flow of life energy and energizes your body. It restores jing that has been lost.

Here is how to practice it:

Stand barefoot in the center of a room with no obstacles around you. Then begin to shake your hands, your arms, your torso, abdomen, pelvis, hips, legs, shoulders, neck, head, and every other part of your body with complete abandon. Do not hold back as you shake, jiggle, wiggle, move, dance, and grind every inch of your body. Let go of everything you have been holding back. Along with the shaking, you might feel like vocalizing. Allow yourself to grunt, sigh, cry, scream, and yell as you let go of all stuck emotions. Continue to do this process until you feel completely loosened and free from shackles and boundaries. Practice this about ten minutes.

When you sense the process is complete, simply stand in one place and take several long, deep, soothing, purifying breaths. Come back to inward and outward balance, and then say the following affirmation audibly, with conviction:

I AM in control. I AM one with Spirit. I AM the only authority in my life. I AM divinely protected by the light of my being. I close off my aura and body of light to the lower astral levels of mind, and I open to the spiritual world. Thank you God, and SO IT IS.

RESTORING HEALTH AND WELL-BEING

When HSP symptoms or physical illness tire or drain you, breathing exercises can restore your vital energy, renew your strength, and bestow robust health. You may record the instructions for this exercise on your device in a soft, slow, soothing voice and then play back the recording when you are ready to practice it.

Lie down on your back on a mat or a bed, and completely relax. Rest your hands lightly over your solar plexus, just above your navel. Breathe slowly, deeply, and smoothly for a few minutes . . . [Record two minutes of silence here.]

Then imagine that with each inhale, you are drawing an increased supply of vital energy, also known as chi or prana, from the infinite universal supply . . . See this inrushing chi being absorbed by your lungs and stored in your navel chakra . . . With every exhale, visualize that energy being distributed all over your body, to every organ . . . muscle . . . cell . . . atom . . . nerve . . . artery . . . and vein . . . from the top of your head to your fingertips, soles of feet, and toes. Continue this process for a few moments . . . [Record one minute of silence here.]

Now continue to visualize inhaling vital life energy and storing it in your navel chakra. And with each exhale, see this life energy invigorating and stimulating every chakra, sending energy and strength throughout your system. Imagine this energy invigorating these areas as you simply place your attention on them, without straining . . . your root chakra . . . pelvic chakra . . . navel chakra . . . heart chakra . . . throat chakra . . . brow chakra . . . and crown chakra . . .

After you feel the distribution of life energy to all parts of your body is complete, then begin to heal your body with your breath. Breathe in deeply as you imagine absorbing a great deal of life force energy . . . As you exhale, visualize sending that energy to an ailing area of your body to stimulate and heal it . . . Then again inhale tremendous life energy . . . Then as you exhale, imagine the diseased condition being expelled from your body . . . Continue this process for a few minutes . . . [Record three minutes of silence here.]

Place both hands over the ill or uncomfortable portion of your body. As you inhale, continue to store life energy in your navel, and with each exhale, imagine life energy flowing down your arms, through your fingertips and palms, into your body . . . Without straining, gently hold the mental image that as you exhale, life energy is pumped into your body through your hands . . . Imagine this energy stimulating your cells, driving out disease . . . Now continue this process for a few minutes . . . [Record three minutes of silence here.]

Then repeat these affirmations audibly, with conviction:

I AM filled with . . . the life force energy in breath . . .
Life energy is healing and lifting . . . any seeming disease from
my body . . .
Life energy is pervading . . . and saturating my body now . . .
I AM healed, strengthened, and invigorated . . . by the power of
life energy now . . . My body is filled with life energy, divine light
. . . divine healing, and divine power now . . .
Thank you God, and SO IT IS.

HEALING ENERGY INVOCATION

The *Siri Gayatri* mantra promotes healing energy and is believed to create a connection with both the earth and the universe, as it allows healing energy to be directed toward another person or location. Please learn how to pronounce it by searching on the Arex YouTube channel for a video named "Snatam Kaur – Ra Ma Da Sa."

Ra Ma Da Sa Sa Say So Hung

This mantra is translated as "Sun, Moon, Earth, Infinity: All that is in infinity, I AM That." Syllables in this mantra are believed to awaken kundalini (spiritual life energy) and direct it up through the spinal column, activating the chakras.

To meditate with this mantra, sit in a comfortable position such as cross-legged or seated on a couch. Bend your elbows and tuck them close to your sides. Extend your forearms away from your body at a 45-degree angle. Open your palms and face them skyward with your fingers together and your thumbs separated. Then chant the mantra Ra Ma Da Sa Sa Say So Hung while placing your attention on each energy center associated with every letter. The syllable sounds and the associated chakras are:

- *Ra (sun)—root chakra*

- *Ma (moon)—sacral chakra*

- *Da (earth)—navel chakra*

- *Sa (impersonal infinity)—heart and throat chakras*

- *Say (totality of infinity)—third eye chakra*

- *So (identity and merger)—crown chakra*

- *Hung (the infinite)—sends energy from the crown back to the root chakra*

"I AM HEALTH" VISUALIZATION

Please record this meditation onto your device in a soft, slow, soothing voice, and then play it back at low volume.

Please sit comfortably and repeat audibly, "I AM health." Then close your eyes. Be absolutely silent and still. Imagine in your mind's eye an intense, magnificent, splendorous, divine light. This light is drawing nearer and nearer to you. It is becoming increasingly bright. As it draws closer, it is so big, bright, and radiant that it nearly blinds you. You can feel this light flooding you from head to toe. Feel the healing warmth of this light. It is so hot that you feel your body perspiring as it burns off all impurities. Continue seeing and feeling this light for a few moments . . . [Record 15 seconds of silence here.] Repeat audibly after me: I AM health . . . I AM health . . . I AM health . . .

Now come forth from this meditation with gratitude by pretending to blow out four candles. Then open your eyes and repeat this affirmation:

I AM alert . . . I AM awake . . . I AM in control . . . I AM divinely protected . . . by the light of my being . . . I AM health . . . I AM health . . . I AM health . . . Thank you God, and SO IT IS.

REMOVING OBSTACLES TO SUCCESS

This is an invocation to Lord Ganesha to remove obstacles and bless your endeavors with prosperity. At the beginning of all undertakings, praying to Lord Ganesha can help, as he is the deity that removes obstacles.[1] You may learn the pronunciation of this chant by searching the Spiritual India YouTube channel under the name "Vakratunda Mahakaya Suryakoti Samaprabha I Ganesh Mantra."

Vakratunda Mahakaya Surya Koti Sama Prabha
Nirvighnam Kuru Me Deva Sarva Karyesu Sarvada

Here is the translation:

O Lord with curved trunk, one with massive body, one with the radiance of ten million Suns, please make all my actions free from troubles.

LOVING MONEY

Why do some people magnetize money like iron filings, yet others constantly complain about being broke? I believe it is because some people love money and others hate it. If you believe "money is the root of all evil," the idea of wealth might repulse you. If you believe "it is easier for a camel to go through the eye of a needle than for a rich man to enter into the kingdom of God," or "blessed are the poor," then you will remain in poverty. If you believe it is wrong to charge money for offering spiritual work, you will always struggle to pay your bills.

These misinterpretations of the Bible have caused millions to be financially destitute and entire nations to be constantly in debt. This meditation can help you attract wealth by developing a love for money. Please record this meditation onto your device in a soft, slow, soothing voice, and then play it back at low volume.

Please sit comfortably and close your eyes. Keep your eyes closed until I tell you to open them. Let us take a big deep breath of relaxation. Breathe in . . . And out . . . Let us take a big deep breath of divine love. Breathe in . . . And out . . . Let us take a big deep breath of inner peace. Breathe in . . . And out . . . Then breathe normally.

We now know that there is one power and one presence in the universe and in our lives, the divine Spirit—omnipresent and omnipotent. Spirit is the source of all substance and supply out of which this universe is made. Spirit is the source of all good. Spirit is good, very good perfection now. Spirit is the source of money, wealth, and riches. This divine source is available for everyone to tap into anytime.

We are now one with Spirit in a complete and perfect wholeness and oneness. There is no separation between ourselves and Spirit. We are fully aligned with and unified with Spirit. There is only one and one only. There is no division. We are merged with that divine source and supply of everything. We are good, very good perfection now. We are the source of money, wealth, and riches. That divine source is at our command, and we can tap into it anytime.

We now therefore know and claim that wealth, riches, money, supply, and all good flows into your life now, with divine order and timing. You now embrace divine bounty and infinite riches without reserve or resistance. You now love money, and money loves you. Money comes to you often and it stays with you always.

We now call upon Spirit to release from your mind all negative beliefs, habits, and patterns about money. You now let go of all false beliefs about money. You release the idea that money is the root of all evil. You let go of the belief that it is easier for a camel to go through the eye of a needle than for a rich man to enter into the kingdom of God. You now dissolve the concept that the poor are blessed and more spiritual than the wealthy. You let go of deep-seated, unconscious jealousy toward wealthy people. You now give up the idea that you hate money because money is bad, money is unspiritual, money will lead you astray, money is undesirable, money is dirty, money can only come through nefarious means, money creates sinful consequences, and money is not of God. All these negative thoughts are lovingly healed, lifted, released, dissolved, and let go now. They are burnt in the fire of divine love. And they are gone.

We now know that you embrace potent, powerful, positive new thoughts and emotions about money. You now know that anyone can tap into the divine source of abundance, simply by asking. You know that money is simply the exchange of energy and it represents goods, services, and assets. You now admire honorable, trustworthy, successful, wealthy people as role models, rather than resenting them. You know that unlimited bounty and supply is available for everyone, money can be used for beneficial purposes, money is spiritual, wealthy people can be blessed and experience divine grace, money is divine, and money is of God. You now love money, and money loves you. It comes to you often and it stays with you permanently. Money is your friend and companion, and you now utilize it for good.

Now take a big deep breath. Breathe in . . . And out . . . Then breathe normally. Now take a moment to visualize what you will do with the wealth you acquire. Paint a vivid picture in your mind's eye of what you plan to create in your life that will necessitate acquiring wealth. By making a clear mental picture, you now magnetize money and draw it into your life. Wealth is never about money for its own sake. It is about using money for good, to manifest your heart's desires, create your most noble dreams, and fulfill your personal mission. As you visualize your goal, place yourself clearly in that situation. Experience that place and see, hear, feel, smell, and taste what is around you . . . [Record one minute of silence here.]

Now, to increase the emotional connection with fulfilling your dream, imagine how you would feel after attaining your goal. Feel deeply the emotions of joy, contentment, satisfaction, security, peace of mind, and all other feelings you would imagine when you have reached your goal. Those feelings will connect you to your desired aspiration and make it real. Spend a few moments feeling these emotions now . . . [Record one minute of silence here.]

Now, with gratitude in your heart, come forth from this meditation and return to objective and subjective balance. Now take deep vigorous breaths and pretend to blow out at least four candles . . . [Record 10 seconds of silence here.] Then open your eyes and repeat the following affirmation with conviction:

I AM alert . . . I AM awake . . . I AM in control . . . I am divinely protected . . . by the light of my being . . . I love money and money loves me . . . It comes to me often . . . and it stays with me permanently . . . Thank you God, and SO IT IS.

WELCOMING WEALTH

Lakshmi (a.k.a. Mahalakshmi) is the Hindu Goddess of abundance, prosperity, wealth (spiritual and material), fortune, and the embodiment of beauty. She is the source and bestower of material contentment and fulfillment. Lakshmi is said to bring good luck and to protect her devotees from money-related problems.

Repeating this powerful Lakshmi mantra produces a vibration that magnetically attracts fortune. The *bija* (seed) mantra *shring* is considered the origin of all powers of the Goddess Lakshmi. Combining it with other sounds forms various mantras. Chant the following mantra at least 108 times, or repeat it in your mind during meditation.[2] You can learn how to pronounce it on the YouTube channel Magical Blessings by searching for "Lakshmi Beej Mantra for Money, Wealth And Happiness."

Om Shring Shriye Namah

Part IV

Rooted in Spiritual Authenticity

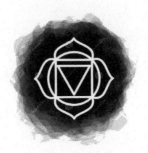

Chapter 10

Living Your Truth

This chapter can help you to live in the moment as your true Self, to dwell in wholeness, and to deal with others with integrity.

GREAT SPIRIT PRAYER

This beautiful Native American prayer of humility expresses the quality of soul that comes from knowing your proper place in the divine order. To gain its benefit, speak this prayer audibly with feeling and conviction:

Oh, Great Spirit, whose voice I hear in the wind, whose breath gives life to all the world.

Hear me; I need your strength and wisdom.

Let me walk in beauty, and make my eyes ever behold the red and purple sunset.

Make my hands respect the things you have made and my ears sharp to hear your voice.

Make me wise so that I may understand the things you have taught my people.

Help me to remain calm and strong in the face of all that comes toward me.

Let me learn the lessons you have hidden in every leaf and rock.

Help me seek pure thoughts and act with the intention of helping others.

Help me find compassion without empathy overwhelming me.

I seek strength, not to be greater than my brother, but to fight my greatest enemy, Myself.

Make me always ready to come to you with clean hands and straight eyes.

So when life fades, as the fading sunset, my spirit may come to
you without shame.

—Translated by Lakota (Sioux) Chief Yellow Lark, 1887

RECLAIMING YOUR INTEGRITY

This affirmation can help you be yourself and live with integrity, free from negative external influences. Please repeat it in a clear voice, with conviction.

I AM the resurrection and the life.
I AM perfection everywhere now.
I AM perfection here now.
I AM free from all negative influences.
I AM pure, integrated, whole, and complete.
Vicissitudes of life may come and go.
But my higher self is unassailable and imperishable.
Nothing can assail my unassailable beingness.
I AM anchored in Spirit.
I AM never wavering, and always true.
I live in truth, and I communicate in truth.
I live in integrity and I attract integrity.
My relationships are in integrity, now and always.
Thank you God, and SO IT IS.

REALIZING YOUR SPIRIT SELF

This meditation can help you embrace your true self—a magnificent being of light, filled with glory, blessedness, and grace. Please read these words onto your device in a soft, slow, soothing voice. Then play back the recording when you are ready to practice it.

Please sit comfortably and close your eyes. Keep your eyes closed until I tell you to open them. Peace, peace, be still. Be still and be at peace. Perfect peace, perfect peace, perfect peace. Be still and be at peace. We now know that God is spiritual awakening and enlightenment. God is wholeness and oneness. God is the ultimate truth and ultimate reality. God is illumination, wisdom, and realization. God is perfection everywhere now. God is perfection here now.

We are now one with, merged with, united with, and fully aligned and allied with God. There is no separation between ourselves and God. For we live, breathe, move, and have our being in God and through God. Therefore we are the wholeness and oneness, the truth and reality, and the illumination and realization that God is. We are spiritual awakening and enlightenment. We are perfection everywhere now. We are perfection here now.

We therefore know and claim that you now realize your own divine nature and your true higher self. Let us take some deep breaths to go deeper. Breathe in . . . And let go . . . Deeper, deeper, deeper, into the wells of Spirit. Let us take a deep breath of inner peace. Breathe in . . . And out . . . Take a big deep breath of relaxation. Breathe in . . . And out . . . Then breathe normally. Peace, peace, be still. Be still and be at peace. Let go, let go, let go, let go, let go, let go, let God. Now take a big deep breath to go deeper. Breathe in . . . And out . . . Then breathe normally. Deeper, deeper, deeper, into the wells of Spirit, into the silence of being. Peace, peace, be at peace. Be still and be at peace.

Now settle down to a place of perfect peace and relaxation. Enter your own sanctum sanctorum within. Draw your attention inward, like a tortoise draws its limbs into its shell. Let yourself become centered, serene, and still. Take another deep breath to go deeper . . . Breathe in . . . And out . . . Then breathe normally. Peace, peace, be still. Be still and be at peace. Perfect peace, perfect peace, perfect peace. Be still and be at peace. Deeper, deeper, deeper, into the wells of Spirit, into the silence of being. We now call upon Holy Spirit to lift you to a higher vibration and to show you your own divine nature. Take a big deep breath. Breathe in . . . And breathe out . . . Then breathe normally.

Now settle down to complete stillness, deep relaxation, and inner peace. Your body is at peace. Your heart rate becomes quiet. Your breath rate is quiet. Your entire body settles down to perfect tranquility. Your conscious mind is perfectly still, like the quietude of the desert at twilight. Your subconscious mind is deep and serene, like the water at the bottom of a well. Now let go of the mind and body. Let yourself merge with Spirit. Allow your awareness to expand to infinite peace, perfect relaxation, wholeness, and oneness. Let go of all vestiges of individuality as you merge fully with absolute bliss consciousness . . . [Record 30 seconds of silence here.]

Know that this wholeness of being is the divine presence within you. This pure contentment is your own true nature. You are the radiant light of Spirit. You are absolute pure consciousness. *Aham Brahmasmi:* I AM that. Thou art that. All this is that. That alone is. Know your self to be that brilliant divine energy. You are a magnificent being of light, blazing with splendor. If you could see yourself as who you really are, you would bow at your own feet. For you are the breath of God. That is who you really are.

With gratitude in your heart, now come forth from this meditation. Take deep vigorous breaths and pretend to blow out four candles . . . [Record 10 seconds of silence here.] Then open your eyes and repeat this affirmation in a strong voice, with conviction:

I AM alert . . . I AM very alert . . . I AM awake . . . I AM very awake . . . I AM inwardly and outwardly balanced . . . I AM divinely protected . . . by the light of my being . . . Thank you God, and SO IT IS.

REALIZING SPIRITUAL ENLIGHTENMENT

Asatoma Sadgamaya is a *shanti* mantra (mantra of peace). It is found in the ancient scripture Brihadaranyaka Upanishads (1.3.28). In Indian schools it is chanted as a prayer during spiritual or religious occasions, social events, and other gatherings. Please learn how to pronounce it by searching the Geethanjali YouTube channel for "Om Asathoma Sadgamaya- Shanti Mantra."

Asato maa sadgamaya
Tamaso maa jyotir gamaya
Mrityor maa amritam gamaya
Sarvesham svastir bhavatu
Sarveshaam shantir bhavatu
Sarveshaam purnam bhavatu
Sarveshaam mangalam bhavatu
Loka samasta sukhino bhavantu
OM shanti, shanti, shanti

Here is the translation:

From ignorance, lead me to truth.
From darkness, lead me to light.
From death, lead me to immortality.
May there be happiness in all.

May there be peace in all.
May there be completeness in all.
May there be success in all.
May all beings everywhere be happy, free, and content.
OM peace, peace, peace.

FULLNESS INVOCATION

This is the mantra of peace (shanti mantra) of the ancient Indian scripture Isha Upanishad (IshaVasya Upanishad), which is a part of the Shukla Yajurveda.[1] Speak this audibly with conviction in order to affirm contentment, fulfillment, oneness, and wholeness. Please learn how to pronounce the mantra by searching the Lata Favs YouTube channel for "Om Poornamadah Poornamidam w/Meaning."

OM poornamadah poornamidam
Poornaat poornamudachyate
Poornasya poornam aadaaya
Poornam eva avashishshyate
OM shaantih shaantih shaantih

Here is the translation:

OM. That is full. This is full,
From the fullness comes the fullness.

If fullness is taken away from fullness,
Only fullness remains.
OM, Peace, peace, peace.

MAHAVATAR BABAJI GAYATRI MANTRA

Here is a mantra to invoke the great sage and guru of gurus, the immortal ascended master, Babaji, who can create miracles in your life. You may read more about this divine master in my book *Ascension.* Learn how to pronounce the mantra by searching the Shivanandi Adi YouTube channel for "Mahavatar Babaji-Mantra Meditation-Babaji Mantra."

*Om Mahavatara Vidmahe
Sat Gurudevaya Deemahi
Tanno Babaji Prachodayat*

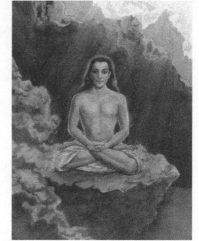

Chapter 11

Fulfilling Your Destiny

This chapter will help you begin to discover, live, and fulfill your true purpose and reach your full potential.

"I AM THE MASTER OF MY DESTINY" AFFIRMATION

At every moment, you have the power to take control of your life. Because you have free will, your every choice in every moment determines your destiny. To gain greater conscious command of your future, you may say this affirmation audibly in a clear voice, with conviction.

I AM the master of my destiny. I AM the captain of my ship.
No one and nothing steers my rudder except me.

I AM in command of my life. I AM the creator of my fate.
I choose to live in the presence of God.
I choose to be of service to humanity.
I choose to be in the world but not of the world.
I choose to be my very best self, my natural self.
I choose to be who I really AM.
I choose to live without fear.
Nothing can diminish my divine presence,
Which is whole, complete, and unassailable.
I AM a mighty, magnificent being of light.
I live in the heart of divine love.
I dwell in the sanctuary of the most high.
I live in the world but I AM of God.

DISCOVERING YOUR TRUE PURPOSE

You were not thrown upon this planet arbitrarily. You have incarnated to fulfill your calling. This meditation can help you discover your life-plan, purpose, and mission. Please read these words onto your device in a soft, slow, soothing voice and then play back the recording.

Please sit comfortably and close your eyes. Keep your eyes closed until I tell you to open them. Let us take a big deep breath of inner peace. Breathe in . . . And out . . . Take a big deep breath of divine love. Breathe in . . . And out . . . Take a big deep breath of relaxation. Breathe in . . . And out . . . Then breathe normally. Peace, peace, be still. Be still and be at peace. Perfect peace, perfect peace, perfect peace. Be still and be at peace.

We now know and recognize that God is our divine mentor. God is our divine guide and counselor, the wayshower on our pathway. God is the lighthouse of our life. God is true purpose, mission, and divine destiny. God is perfection everywhere now. God is perfection here now. We are now merged with and one with God in a perfect seamless wholeness. There is no separation between ourselves and God. We are the divine mentor and counselor that God is. We are the wayshower and lighthouse that guides our pathway. We are divine purpose, mission, and destiny. We now therefore know and claim that you now uncover and fulfill the true plan and purpose of your life.

You now let go of any and all beliefs, habits, emotions, conditions, and influences that have blocked you from fulfilling your purpose. You now release, dissolve, lift, and let go of any and all thoughts of fear of failure, jealousy of those you admire, resentment about bad luck, shame about compromising your values, guilt about not following your heart, blame toward those who held you back— and feeling undeserving of success, regret about time wasted, and lack of financial prosperity. These thoughts are now lifted, loved, healed, dissolved, released, and let go into the divine light of truth. And they are gone.

You now welcome and accept into your life new, powerful, positive thoughts and emotions of faith, trust, success, self-love, self-worth, self-confidence, goodwill and good wishes toward successful people, letting go of past failures, a positive attitude toward the future, deserving success, forgiving your seeming mistakes, forgiving compromising your values, forgiving indulging in regret, courage to follow your heart, forgiving people who held you back, realizing the past cannot be changed, realizing time is never wasted and every drop of effort is precious, and accepting and welcoming financial prosperity. These positive thoughts manifest in your mind now.

Peace, peace, be still. Be still and be at peace. Perfect peace, perfect peace, perfect peace. Be still and be at peace. Now take a deep breath to go deeper into meditation. Breathe in . . . And out . . . Take a deep breath to go even deeper. Breathe in . . . And out . . . Then breathe normally. Now get quiet, still, and centered within your heart. Allow yourself to be still, quiet, and peaceful. Take another deep breath to go deeper. Breathe in . . . And out . . . Then breathe normally. Let go, let go, let go, let go, let go, let go, let God. Now settle down to a state of pure relaxation and contentment. You are now at peace.

Now, within your heart, and also audibly, you will ask a question of Spirit. You will then take a big deep breath and afterwards do what I call the "do-nothing program." That means do nothing, nothing, and less than nothing. Do not seek or force an answer to your question. Let go of all expectations. Simply be quiet, get still, have a neutral attitude, and be open to receive. The answer will come to you as an inner vision, voice, or feeling.

Now is time to ask your question of Spirit. Here is the question to ask: "What is my divine purpose and mission for this lifetime?" Please ask the question verbally now . . . Then breathe in . . . And out . . . Then breathe normally and do the do-nothing program. Allow yourself plenty of time to receive the answer. Breathe in . . . And out . . . [Record two minutes of silence here.]

Now, with gratitude in your heart, it is time to return from the meditation and come back to inward and outward balance. Please pretend you are blowing out at least four candles . . . [Record 10 seconds of silence here.] Then say this affirmation with eyes wide open:

I AM alert . . . I AM very alert . . . I AM awake . . . I AM very awake . . . I AM in control . . . I AM the only authority in my life . . . I AM divinely protected . . . by the light of my being . . . Thank you God, and SO IT IS.

AFFIRMATION OF GRACE

To welcome the miracle-making power of divine grace into your life, speak this affirmation audibly, with firm conviction. To learn more about the Law of Grace, please read my book *Miracle Prayer*.

The Law of Grace is at work in my life now
Annihilating karmic law and replacing it
With perfection everywhere now.
I AM united, merged, and one with Spirit now.
I AM an instrument of Spirit's love, light, and peace.
I AM perfection everywhere now.
I AM perfection here now.
I claim my good, very good perfection now.
Thank you God, and SO IT IS.

LIVING YOUR POTENTIAL

If you feel you are not fulfilling your potential, this affirmation can help you to let go of limitations and manifest your destiny. Speak this audibly in a strong, powerful voice with conviction:

I now see, know, and accept that I have the power to do anything
I set my mind to. There are no limitations. I AM free from old
habits, beliefs, and conditioning that have a stranglehold on me.

I call upon Spirit to now release from my energy field any and all old encrusted armors that have blocked me from achieving my goals. I now lovingly crack open, crumble up, dissolve, heal, lift, release, and let go of all façade bodies and belief bodies of limitation, reticence, and fear of fulfilling my true potential. I AM in control. I AM the only authority in my life. I AM divinely protected by the light of my being. I now renew my enthusiasm and resolve to fulfill my true potential. I AM now determined to do whatever it takes to realize my divine destiny in this lifetime. Thank you God, and SO IT IS.

GAYATRI MANTRA OR SAVITRI MANTRA

Gayatri Mantra is a hymn from the ancient Indian scripture RigVeda (10:16:3). Attributed to sage Vishwaamitra, the mantra is directed toward Goddess Gayatri, who is not considered a deity, but the one supreme personality.

Spiritual aspirants recite Gayatri to remember their higher purpose, to invoke the Supreme, to attain higher consciousness, and to know the ultimate truth. It is traditional to chant this mantra 108 times. Please learn how to pronounce it by searching the Shemaroo Bhakti YouTube channel for "Gayatri Mantra 108 Times Chanting | Om Bhur Bhuva Swaha."

Aum Bhoor Bhuvah Swaha,
Tat Savitur Varenyam
Bhargo Devasaya Dheemahi
Dhiyo Yo Naha Prachodayat

Here is the translation:

Oh Supreme one; which is the physical, astral and causal worlds itself. You are the source of all, deserving all worship. Radiant, divine one; we meditate upon you. Propel our intellect toward liberation.[1]

Chapter 12

Making a Positive Influence

Your every thought, word, and deed is influencing not only you, but the entire universe. You can amplify your positive effect on the atmosphere by practicing the methods in this chapter. More specific affirmations for healing the earth and restoring ecological balance can be found in my book *Third Eye Meditations*.

CLEARING THE ATMOSPHERE

Have you ever entered a building and immediately felt you were punched in the stomach with its exceedingly dense vibrational atmosphere? This is common in old buildings, prisons, mental institutions, schools, hospitals, bars, and private homes where residents have been arguing, or where earthbound spirits are hanging on.

It is easy to eliminate negative atmospheric vibrations. Even a haunted building can be transformed into a heavenly space. Just speak the following affirmation audibly in a strong voice:

All negative vibrations and earthbound spirits that are in this building are now lovingly healed and forgiven, healed and forgiven, healed and forgiven, healed and forgiven, healed and forgiven, lifted in love, and united with the truth of being. You are filled, surrounded, and pervaded with divine love and light. Fear, pain, and the earthly vibration no longer bind you. You are now free from all lower vibrations.

You are now lifted into the light of Spirit, lifted into the light of Spirit, lifted into the light of Spirit. You are free to move on into the light and to go to your perfect place of expression. You are bless-ed, forgiven, and released into the love, light, and wholeness of universal Spirit. You are bless-ed, forgiven, and released into the love, light, and wholeness of universal Spirit. You are bless-ed, forgiven, and released into the love, light, and wholeness of universal Spirit. You are lifted into the light of God. Go now in love. Go now in peace.

I now call upon the Holy Spirit to shine the light of truth upon this building now and to fill and surround this building with the pure white light and white fire of Spirit. I now call upon

Master Jesus to build a beautiful golden sphere of divine light and to encase this building in that sphere. The golden, glittering Christ light now fills and surrounds this sphere, lifting the vibration of this building to the Christ consciousness energy or better. I call upon Archangel Michael to stand sentry above, below, and on every side of this sphere, waving his blue flame sword of truth, bringing divine protection and divine will. Any astral entities that need healing are now healed at the outer edge of this sphere.

I call forth Saint Germain to pervade this building with the violet purifying flame, to lift the vibration of this building to ascension vibration or better. I call forth Mahamuni Babaji to fill this space with the clear light of spiritual enlightenment, to illuminate this building with the radiance of the Himalayan saints and siddhas [perfected beings] of India. I call forth Mother Mary and Kwan Yin to fill this space with the pure pink light of divine unconditional love and compassion.

I now call upon the angels and archangels of God to encircle this building and feed it with divine love and light. I call upon all the divine beings who come in the name of God and who are guardians of this building to come forth and feed the building with divine grace and blessings. I now know this building is free from negative energy, which is now lifted, healed, released, let go, and burnt in the fire of divine love. All these divine light beings are now beaming and blazing divine light into this building, lifting, lifting, lifting, lifting, lifting, lifting, lifting the energy of this building into the vibration of divine love. I now thank God for manifesting the healing of this building, and I know this building is blessed with divine love and light. Thank you God, and SO IT IS.

AFFIRMATION OF IDEAL BEHAVIOR

This affirmation, composed by Bahá'u'lláh of the Baha'i religion, and revised for use as a self-empowering declaration, can inspire you to be a positive influence for yourself, your family, friends, and society at large. Repeat it audibly with strength and conviction:

I AM generous in prosperity, and thankful in adversity.

I AM fair in my judgment, and guarded in my speech.

I AM a lamp unto those who walk in darkness, and a home to the stranger.

I AM eyes to the blind, and a guiding light unto the feet of the erring.

I AM a breath of life to the body of humankind,

A dew to the soil of the human heart,

And a fruit upon the tree of humility.

"THE FOUR IMMEASURABLES" OF BUDDHA

Buddha believed meditation could cultivate loving kindness, compassion, happiness, and equanimity for all beings. These "Four Immeasurables" affect immeasurable beings with immeasurably positive results. These sublime states of mind mirror the mind of God. Speak this affirmation audibly with conviction:

May all sentient beings have happiness and the causes of happiness.

May all sentient beings be free from suffering and the causes of suffering.

May all sentient beings never be separated from the happiness that is without suffering.

May all sentient beings abide in equanimity, free from both attachment and hatred, holding some close and others distant.[1]

AFFIRMATION TO RELIEVE SUFFERING

This affirmation of compassion can relieve the suffering of all beings. It was written by Buddha. Repeat this audibly with strength and conviction:

May all beings everywhere plagued with sufferings of body and mind quickly be freed from their illnesses.

May those frightened cease to be afraid, and may those bound be free.

May the powerless find power, and may people think of befriending one another.

May those who find themselves in trackless, fearful wilderness— the children, the aged, the unprotected—be guarded by beneficent celestials, and may they swiftly attain enlightenment.

COMPASSION FOR ALL BEINGS

This Buddhist prayer is a clarion call for all beings to live in love and joy. Say it audibly with deep feeling and conviction:

> *May all beings everywhere,*
> *Both seen and unseen,*
> *Dwelling far off or nearby,*
> *Being, or waiting to become:*
> *May all be filled with lasting joy.*
> *Let no one deceive another,*
> *Let no one anywhere despise another,*
> *Let no one out of anger or resentment*
> *Wish suffering to anyone at all.*
> *Just as a mother with her own life*
> *Protects her child, her only child, from hurt,*
> *So within ourselves let grow*
> *A boundless love for all creatures.*
> *Let our love flow out through the whole universe*
> *To its full height, depth, and broad extent,*
> *Then, as we stand or walk, sit or lie down,*
> *As long as we are awake,*
> *Let us strive for this with a one-pointed mind.*
> *Our life will bring heaven to earth.*

PROTECTION AND WELL-BEING OF HUMANITY

This mantra may be chanted as an offering of loving-kindness to all beings, including yourself. The origin of this mantra is from the Brhadaranyaka Upanishad, though not in its present form.[2] To learn the proper pronunciation, please search the Purple Valley Ashtanga Yoga YouTube channel for "Ashtanga Yoga Closing Mantra."

Om. Svasti prajabhyah paripalayantam nyayena margena mahim mahishah

Gobrahmanebhyah shubham astu nityam lokah samastah sukhino bhavantu

Here is the translation:

May the rulers of the earth protect the well-being of the people
With justice, by means of the right path.
May there always be good fortune for all living beings.
May all beings in the world be full of happiness and free.
May our thoughts, our words, and our actions contribute to that happiness and freedom.

SHANTI MANTRA

This Peace Mantra is taken from Krishna Yajurveda Taittiriya Upanishad (2.2.2). It is often recited in schools as prayer before classes start.[3] Learn how to pronounce it by searching the Geethanjali YouTube channel for "Om Sahana Vavatu | Shanti Mantra | With Lyrics And Meaning."

OM saha naavavatu
Saha nau bhunaktu
Saha veeryam karavaavahai
Tejasvi naavadheetamastu
Maa vidvishaavahai
OM shaantih, shaantih, shaantih

Here is the translation:

OM, May we all be protected.
May we all be nourished.
May we work together with great energy.
May our intellect be sharpened (may our study be effective).
Let there be no animosity amongst us.
OM, peace (in me), peace (in nature), peace (in divine forces).

PEACE CHANT

This chant is used in India at the end of many ceremonies and prayers.

OM shaantih, shaantih, shaantih

Translation:

I invoke the supreme energy of creation to create peace for all beings.

Part V

Rooted in Spiritual Awakening

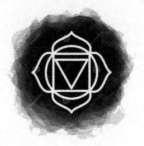

Chapter 13

Jump-Starting Primal Energy

Earth energies are primarily located in the root chakra, which is the home of the spiritual life-force energy known as kundalini. This chapter will introduce methods for waking up kundalini, increasing your energy, and lifting your awareness. To learn more about kundalini energy, please read my book *The Big Book of Chakras and Chakra Healing*.

WAKING UP KUNDALINI

Here are four mantras that wake up kundalini where it is sleeping in the "root bulb" of muladhara (root chakra). These mantras increase sexual attraction, passion, and potency; enhance sexual desire; and remove hindrances to the flow of sexual energy. Each of these mantras invokes Kamadeva, who is the deity of love, known in the West as cupid.

The first is Kamdev Gayatri Mantra. You may learn how to pronounce it by searching the Rajshri Soul YouTube channel for "Kamdev Gayatri Mantra 108 Times | Mantra To Get Love in Life." In addition, the *bija* (seed) mantra, *kleeng* can be used independently to jump start the flow of kundalini energy. Just by chanting this mantra, you might feel a surge of sexual stimulation.

Kleeng kamadevaya vidmahe pushpa banaya dheemahi tanno anangah prachodayaat

Translation:

I meditate on Kamdeva, the master of the senses, who wields arrows of flowers. May that *ananga* (one without a body) give me higher intellect and illuminate my mind.

You can learn how to pronounce the second mantra by searching the MusicMagic YouTube channel for "Mantra to Increase Sexual Energy | Kamdev Kameshwari Maha Tantra."

Om namo kamadevaaye mahaprabhaye hrim kameshvari swaha

To learn to pronounce the third mantra, please search the MusicMagic YouTube channel for "kamdev mantra | Om Kleem Kamadevaya Namah | Marriage & Love Mantra."

Om kleem kamadevaya namah

This fourth mantra cannot be located on YouTube, but it might be the most potent of all. It is known as the Kamadeva Vashikaran Mantra. Here is the phonetic spelling of the mantra.

Om Namomi Bhagvataye Kamdevayaye, yasyaa yasyaa drishyo Bhaavami, Yaashch Yaashch mum muukhaam paashyati taammy taammy mohyatu swahaa

KUNDALINI BANDHA

In this section you will learn powerful esoteric exercises from India that help you awaken *kundalini*. They are called *bandha*, which means "muscular lock." Let us learn how to practice them.

Jalandhara Bandha: Throat Lock

Jalandhara bandha is a lock that forces *kundalini* to flow into *sushumna nadi*, the energy passage through which *kundalini* rises up the center of the spinal canal. This simple bandha brings mental balance, tranquility, and introversion. The ancient scriptures claim it can prevent old age and death. Let us learn it now.

Practice this bandha in a comfortable position: cross-legged, sitting on a chair, or standing, with feet close together. If seated, place your palms on your knees. If standing, bend your knees slightly and place your palms on your thighs.

Close your eyes and relax your entire body. Inhale deeply through your nose and then exhale fully as you bend your neck forward and press your chin tightly against the sternal notch. Straighten your arms and lock elbows while holding your knees (if sitting) or thighs (if standing). Locking elbows intensifies the pressure applied to the neck. Simultaneously, hunch your shoulders upward and forward. This keeps your arms straight and elbows locked. Stay in this position and place your attention on your throat area while holding your breath as long as comfortable.

When you need to take a breath, relax your shoulders, slowly raise your head, and inhale slowly. Breathe normally. Repeat this process as many times as comfortable.

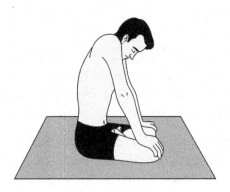

Practice jalandhara bandha before meditation. Do not practice it if you have high blood pressure or heart ailments.

Uddiyana Bandha: Abdominal Lock

Uddiyana (raise up, fly upward) *bandha* causes your diaphragm to rise upward toward your chest. This practice moves kundalini energy upward through the chakras to your crown chakra. The ancient scriptures claim uddiyana bandha is useful for expanding awareness, reversing aging, and attaining immortality.

Practice uddiyana bandha before breakfast in the morning on an empty stomach, after evacuating your bowels.

Practice this bandha in cross-legged or standing position. Let us try it standing, the easiest method. Stand with feet about one and a half feet apart. Bend forward slightly at your waist and bend your legs slightly. Place your palms on your thighs near knees and place pressure on your thighs. Empty your lungs as much as possible by blowing out repeatedly. Bend your neck downward and press your chin against your sternal notch in chin lock (jalandhara bandha).

Then make a false inhalation. That means expand your chest as though breathing in, but contract your throat, preventing air from entering your lungs. Straighten your legs slightly. This raises the diaphragm, and the abdomen takes a concave shape, inward and upward. Hold this position for as long as you can hold your breath.

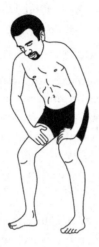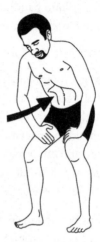

Most people practice this bandha incorrectly by forcing the abdominal muscles to take a concave shape. However, taking a false inhalation automatically raises your diaphragm.

When you can no longer hold your breath, relax your arms, release jalandhara bandha, slowly lift your head, and take a breath. This is one round. Practice several rounds and gradually increase the number of rounds over several weeks. After practicing this in standing position for several months, try it in a seated posture.

Mula Bandha: Perineum Contraction Lock

The Sanskrit term *mula* means base or root. Here it refers to muladhara chakra, seat of kundalini, and also the perineum. Let us learn how to practice it.

While practicing this bandha, the trigger point to be contracted in the male is the perineum between the anus and genitals. In the female, it is the G-Spot or Gräfenberg spot near the cervix. Most people practice moola bandha incorrectly by contracting only the anus.

Practice this bandha in a comfortable seated, cross-legged, or standing position. To strengthen the physical contraction, you may place one heel on your perineum area and apply firm pressure. Close your eyes and relax your entire body. Exhale fully.

Strongly contract your muscles at the trigger point, without excessive strain. Hold your attention at the point of contraction. Remain in the bandha as long as possible while holding your breath. Then let go of the contraction and inhale. This is one round. Practice several more rounds as comfortable.

Moola bandha awakens the root chakra, arouses kundalini to enter the sushumna channel, transmutes sexual energy, maintains prostate health and male potency, and prevents sexual, bladder, and anal incontinence. This bandha balances the dynamic life force energies in the body.

HANG SAH BREATHING

A simple, effective breathing exercise that can relax you deeply is known as Hang Sah breathing. This exercise is performed with mouth slightly open. Here is how:

As you inhale, whisper the mantra "Haaaaaaaang," and as you exhale, whisper "Saaaaaaaaah." Continue this practice for five to ten minutes.

DAKINI MANTRA

Vajrayogini is a dakini ("sky-dancer")—a wild spirit who dances ecstatically in the clear blue sky of emptiness. She is depicted as blood red in color, naked except for ornaments of human bone and a necklace of skulls, corresponding to the letters of the Sanskrit alphabet, and symbolizing purification of speech.

In her right hand she holds a knife, with which she cuts off attachments. In her left hand is a skull cup filled with *mahasukha* (the great bliss), which she pours out like wine to her devotees. In the crook of her left arm is a magic staff.

Chant this mantra to increase your vital energy and to eliminate fear and delusional thinking. To learn how to pronounce the mantra, please go to the YouTube channel for Anil Thapa, Honoring The Land, and search for "Vajrayogini Mantra."

Om om om sarva buddha dakiniye vajra varnaniye vajra
vairocaniye hum hum hum phat phat phat svaha

PANCHAKSHARA MANTRA

Panchakshara literally means "five letters" in Sanskrit and refers to five holy syllables: *Na, Ma, Shi, Vaa* and *Ya*. These five syllables comprise the Panchakshara Mantra, which relates to a prayer to Lord Shiva written by the great Shri Adi Shankaracharya, perhaps the greatest saint of ancient India.

To stimulate vital energy, recite these mantras audibly at the same time as you focus on these chakra points. See the figure on page 162 to help you locate the points:

Naaaaaaaa: Root Chakra

Maaaaaaaa: Sacred Chakra

SHiiiiiiiiiiii: Navel Chakra

Vaaaaaaaa: Heart Chakra

Yaaaaaaaa: Throat Chakra

CHAKRA MANTRAS

You may use the chakra *bija mantras* (one-syllable seed sounds) to stimulate and unblock each chakra. Respectively, each sound aligns with the seven major energy centers: root chakra: *Muladhara,* pelvic chakra: *Svadishthana,* navel chakra: *Manipura,* heart chakra: *Anahata,* throat chakra: *Vishuddha,* brow chakra: *Ajna,* and crown chakra: *Sahasrara.* When you are feeling out of balance in any area of life, it is beneficial to chant these mantras as you place attention on each of the chakras associated with the mantras. See the image on page 162 to locate the chakra points.

Lam: root chakra

Vam: pelvic chakra

Ram: navel chakra

Yam: heart chakra

Ham: throat chakra

Om: brow chakra

Silence: crown chakra

Chapter 14

Firing the Caldron

I n this chapter you will learn the importance of the lower chakras for increasing and expanding life force energy throughout your body. You can use these practices to increase the flow of life energy through your system.

QUICKENING BREATH

The "quickening breath" increases energy circulation throughout your subtle body. Imbibing more vital life energy into your lungs increases inner strength, power, health, happiness, mental clarity, energy, calm, and peace. Whenever you feel tired, angry, weak, or cranky, spend a few minutes practicing this method to revitalize your system. Here is how:

Place your hand on your abdomen. Keep your mouth closed while breathing deeply and quickly through your nose, exhaling and inhaling fully. While inhaling, distend your abdomen. While exhaling, contract it.

Here is a hint: Focus your attention on the exhale. Contract your abdominal muscles with a backward push as you quickly, forcefully exhale. Then your abdomen will naturally distend during inhalation. Repeat at least 10 times.

MICROCOSMIC ORBIT

The "microcosmic orbit" is a Taoist visualization that prevents depletion of your *jing* (primal life essence) resulting from loss of sexual fluids. It circulates and refines *chi* (life force energy) via an energy circuit that runs from your perineum to your head, then back down to your perineum. This practice harmonizes and transmutes the vital fluids and generates vitality.

In this method, the usual downward outlet of jing or essence (to create offspring) is reversed. You will inhale into the lower abdomen at pelvic chakra *(dantian)*, and force *kundalini* (life energy) and jing (generative force) to rise upward from the base of the spine to the top of the head through the "governing vessel" *(dumai:* rear midline channel), which connects all the body's yang meridians, through the chakras along the spine.

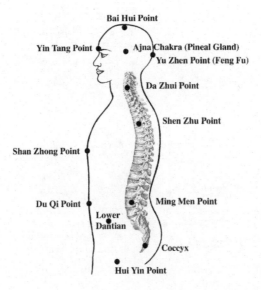

Then you will exhale and relax the lower abdomen, so the kundalini and jing move down the "conception channel" *(renmai:* front midline channel), which connects all the yin meridians, through the chakra trigger points *(kshetram)* along the front of the body.

The orbit runs through the base of the spine *(huiyin:* root chakra*),* up to the coccyx, then to the spot between the kidneys *(mingmen:*

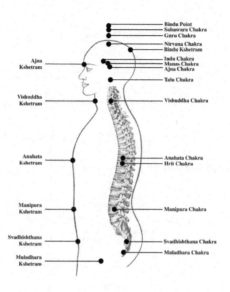

Bindu Point
Sahasrara Chakra
Guru Chakra
Nirvana Chakra
Bindu Kshetram
Indu Chakra
Manas Chakra
Ajna Chakra
Talu Chakra

Ajna
Kshetram

Vishuddha
Kshetram

Vishuddha Chakra

Anahata
Kshetram

Anahata Chakra
Hrit Chakra

Manipura
Kshetram

Manipura Chakra

Svadhishthana
Kshetram

Svadhishthana Chakra

Muladhara
Kshetram

Muladhara Chakra

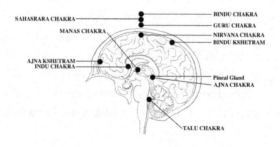

SAHASRARA CHAKRA

BINDU CHAKRA

GURU CHAKRA

MANAS CHAKRA

NIRVANA CHAKRA
BINDU KSHETRAM

AJNA KSHETRAM
INDU CHAKRA

Pineal Gland
AJNA CHAKRA

TALU CHAKRA

navel chakra), to the back of the head (*yuzhen:* rear part of third eye chakra), to the top of the brain *(baihui:* nirvana chakra). Then it flows down the front of the body to the brow chakra *(yintang)*, heart *(shanzhong)*, navel *(duqi)*, and perineum *(huiyin)*. This completes one full rotation of the circuit.

Please record the following meditation onto your device in a soft, gentle voice. Then play back the recording in a low volume.

Sit upright with feet flat on the floor, sitting forward, with only your buttocks on the chair. Close your eyes and focus attention on your lower dantian, about two inches below your navel. Visualize a small, luminous gold or white chi energy ball, bright and pure. Maintain attention on the lower dantian until you feel the ball as heat, vibration, warmth, or sensation . . .

Close your mouth and breathe through your nostrils. As you inhale into your belly, your abdomen will expand. As you exhale, your abdomen will contract. Keep your tongue pressed lightly against the roof of your mouth with the tip of your tongue touching the back of your upper front teeth.

Take a deep breath into the belly and imagine the chi ball moving down from the lower dantian, past the perineum, up the spine to coccyx. Then imagine the ball rising up your spine to the navel point in the spine, then farther up the spine to the back of the head, to the throat chakra point at the neck.

Then imagine this chi ball in the center of your brain, at the pineal gland (crystal palace), absorbing healing energy from baihui (nirvana chakra at top of your brain). Next, focus your attention on the brow chakra at your forehead just above your eyebrows, and draw energy into the chi ball from that third eye point, as the ball passes to the roof of your mouth. You may feel a tingling or throbbing sensation in your mouth. This ends one inhalation.

Then, as you exhale, see the energy ball move down through your palate and tongue (as your tongue is still lightly pressed against your palate), into your throat to the heart point. From the heart, move it down through your solar plexus and down into the lower dantian, where the energy gathers, mixes, and is stored for internal circulation.

Then begin another cycle of inhalation and exhalation. You can practice this orbit several times.

You can use this beneficial meditation sitting during the day or lying down before sleep. If you have trouble imagining the flow, try visualizing a golf ball or Ping-Pong ball. You can even trace the flow with your finger during the practice. For more details about this Taoist meditation, please read my book *Awaken Your Third Eye*, chapter 10.

KUNDALINI RISING

Kundalini arohanam means "kundalini rising." This powerful chant nudges kundalini energy, lying dormant in root chakra, to rise up the spine to the crown chakra above the head. There the feminine Shakti Kundalini energy unites with the masculine Shiva. For more information about chakras and kundalini, please read my book *The Big Book of Chakras and Chakra Healing*.

Three components are involved in this meditative process: awareness, visualization, and sound vibrations. These activate the seven major chakras and open doors of perception, as you connect with inner divinity.

Sit comfortably with back support. Then recite the words while focusing on each chakra. Keep your attention on each separate chakra point as its name and mantras are chanted. While chanting "kundalini arohanam," visualize a bright golden fluid flooding each chakra, turning it to bright golden light.

Please see the figure on page 162 to locate the chakra points. For the correct pronunciation, listen to the chant on the Esencial Natura YouTube channel and search for "Ananda Giri The Oneness Chakra Meditation."

Om muladhara [place attention on root chakra].

Lang, Lang, Lang, Lang, Lang, Lang, Lang.

Om, kundalini arohanam, kundalini arohanam, kundalini arohanam.

Om

Om svadhishthana [place attention on pelvic chakra].

Vang, Vang, Vang, Vang, Vang, Vang, Vang.

Om, kundalini arohanam, kundalini arohanam, kundalini arohanam.

Om

Om manipura [place attention on navel chakra].

Rang, Rang, Rang, Rang, Rang, Rang, Rang.

Om, kundalini arohanam, kundalini arohanam, kundalini arohanam.

Om

Om anahata [place attention on heart chakra].

Yang, Yang, Yang, Yang, Yang, Yang, Yang.

Om, kundalini arohanam, kundalini arohanam, kundalini arohanam.

Om

Om vishuddha [place attention on throat chakra].

Hang, Hang, Hang, Hang, Hang, Hang, Hang.

Om, kundalini arohanam, kundalini arohanam, kundalini arohanam.

Om

Om ajna [place attention on brow chakra].

Aum, Aum, Aum, Aum, Aum, Aum, Aum.

Om, kundalini arohanam, kundalini arohanam, kundalini arohanam.

Om

Om sahasrara [place attention on crown chakra].

Ogum Satyam Om, Ogum Satyam Om, Ogum Satyam Om, Ogum Satyam Om, Ogum Satyam Om, Ogum Satyam Om, Ogum Satyam Om.

Om, kundalini arohanam, kundalini arohanam, kundalini arohanam.

Om

Om mulahara [place attention on root chakra].

Om svadhishthana [place attention on pelvic chakra].

Om manipura [place attention on navel chakra].

Om anahata [place attention on heart chakra].

Om vishuddha [place attention on throat chakra].

Om ajna [place attention on brow chakra].

Om sahasrara [place attention on crown chakra].

Om shantih, shantih, shantih.

Chapter 15

Journeys to Spiritual Vortexes

In this chapter you will enjoy guided visualization journeys to sacred destinations throughout the world. To enjoy these journeys, please read and record them onto your device. Then sit comfortably, close your eyes, and listen to these guided meditations as you follow the instructions step by step.

JOURNEY TO MOUNT SHASTA

Please record this visualization on your device:

Please sit comfortably and close your eyes. Keep your eyes closed until I tell you to open them. Let us take a big deep breath of divine love. Breathe in . . . And out . . . Take a big deep breath of divine light. Breathe in . . . And out . . . And a big deep breath of relaxation. Breathe in . . . And out . . . Then breathe normally.

Let us imagine it is a glorious, sunny day in July. You arrive on Mount Shasta at 7500 feet in the parking area for upper Panther Meadow. It is about 75 degrees Fahrenheit as you head toward the meadow.

Immediately you are struck by the deep silence enveloping the atmosphere. Walking silently along a dirt trail that winds through a grove of red firs, you hear the soothing sound of burbling streams trickling over the landscape. You enter a rolling bright emerald blanket of grass known as Panther Meadow. The meadow is edged with large boulders, and in the distance, a sunbather lies on one of the rocks, enjoying the healing rays of sunlight.

The afternoon sun blazes over the land, and the evergreens cast deep shadows across the grass. This bucolic scene is embellished by an explosion of wildflowers of white, crimson, yellow, violet, gold, blue, pink, and magenta and an orchestra of jaybirds, warblers, and mountain chickadees. As you make your way around the meadow, you stop to lean down and take a refreshing drink from a trickling spring that meanders about the countryside.

You follow the trail up to the area of a pure spring bubbling up from underground. It is surrounded on three sides by a rock wall about five feet tall. Just south of the spring, you fill your water bottle in the babbling brook, and as you drink of this nectar of the Gods you feel entirely renewed, revived, and refreshed.

Suddenly a stranger appears, and you immediately sense that this is no ordinary man. The stranger has deep penetrating eyes, long, shining black hair, and he wears an intricately designed tunic and tight-fitting trousers in the style of 18th century Europe. He approaches you with a friendly smile. He then asks why you have come to his home. As you answer the stranger, you realize this place is not only his home; it is also yours. You have returned to a place so familiar, as though you have lived here for centuries.

The stranger then says, "I will now reveal your divine purpose."

In an instant, you are transported to a glorious temple of marble and inlaid precious and semi-precious gemstones. As you enter the temple, you are ushered into a chamber where you are bathed in a pure crystalline liquid that permeates every pore with healing energies.

You then enter another chamber where pure divine light of every color rotates through the spectrum, penetrating your being with vitality and well-being. At the same time, heavenly celestial music lifts your vibration to a higher energetic octave. After these treatments, you are clothed in an ornately embroidered silken garment, and you enter a chamber where a group of ascended beings hold council.

There you are seated on a golden velvet-cushioned throne encrusted with gemstones. A dozen ascended masters approach you one by one. Each of them bows to you and anoints you with perfumes and oils.

After this healing ritual, you feel completely invigorated. You enter another room where ascended masters are seated at a round table of pure alabaster. As you sit at the table, a discussion begins about what you have accomplished in this lifetime, and what you intend to accomplish going forward. The divine beings give you insights into what your true mission and purpose is, and how you might fulfill it . . . [Record one minute of silence here.]

Once all your questions and concerns are answered by these ascended beings, you now find yourself back on Mount Shasta in the afternoon sun, standing alone next to the spring on Panther Meadow. The anachronistic stranger has vanished.

Now it is time to come forth from this visualization. Give gratitude to Spirit. Then pretend to vigorously blow out a candle as you come forth from the level of Spirit to your subconscious mind, which has been permanently transformed, lifted, and healed by this meditation. Then blow out another candle and affirm that your conscious mind is now one with the divine mind. Blow out a third candle and know that your body is now filled with robust health and energy. Then blow out a fourth candle as you return to this room and this place and time. Know that you are bringing all the blessings of Spirit into your environment.

Finally, blow out four more candles, come out of meditation, and then open your eyes . . . [Record 10 seconds of silence here.] With eyes wide open, now repeat the following affirmation:

I AM alert . . . I AM awake . . . I AM very alert . . . I AM very awake . . . I AM in control . . . I AM the only authority in my life . . . I AM divinely protected . . . by the light of my being . . . Thank you God, and SO IT IS.

JOURNEY TO MACHU PICCHU, PERU

Please record this visualization on your device:

Please sit comfortably and close your eyes. Keep your eyes closed until I tell you to open them. Let us take a big deep breath of divine love. Breathe in . . . And out . . . Take a big deep breath of divine light. Breathe in . . . And out . . . And a big deep breath of relaxation. Breathe in . . . And out . . . Then breathe normally.

Early in the morning, before dawn on the March equinox, the temperature is 60 degrees Fahrenheit and the air is crisp in the mountain town of Aguas Calientes. You board a bus that takes you farther up the mountain. After 25 minutes of switchback roads, you arrive at your cloud-covered mystical destination in the sky: the ancient holy city of Machu Picchu, Peru, at about 8,000 feet elevation.

You walk through a gateway that transports you into another time, place, and dimension. A parade of ancient Inca priests, dressed in colorful costumes, arrives to greet you. They welcome you with music and dancing, and offer you fresh fruits, sweets, gold, and precious gemstones.

There is great jubilation as you enter the sacred grounds. In the predawn glow, the magical splendor of the granite-carved temples, palaces, baths, dwellings, storage rooms, and terraces set upon a verdant mountain of emerald green grasses takes your breath away.

Next you and your Inca guides witness the rising sun at the Temple of the Three Windows, which is aligned to the east. The three windows represent the underground (Uku-Pacha), the heaven (Hanan-Pacha), and the present time (Kay-Pacha). As the sun rises, your guides perform an ancient ritual of thanksgiving . . . [Record 20 seconds of silence here.]

You continue your journey to the Principle Temple, where building blocks weighing more than 50 tons are sculpted and fitted together with no mortar and with such precision that the joints do not allow even a thin knife blade to be inserted. There, dancing and celebration takes place, and a great breakfast feast is served . . . [Record 10 seconds of silence here.]

Next, enter the sacred springs of the Ritual Fountains, where your Inca guides anoint you with holy waters. You imbibe the pristine waters and then rest at the nearby Temple of the Sun. As you enter a deep, entrancing meditation, you are given keys that unlock the ancient mysteries embedded in these granite stones . . . [Record 30 seconds of silence here.]

Now your Inca guides lead you to an unusual-shaped granite rock—an astronomical observatory known as Intihuatana, the "Hitching Post of the Sun," for an equinox ritual. It is believed this stone is designed to "hitch the sun" at the two equinoxes. At midday, the sun stands directly above the pillar, casting no shadow whatsoever. The sun "sits with all his might upon the pillar" and is for a moment "tied" to the rock. Your Inca guides encircle the stone, chant in an ancient language, and perform a ritual to "tie the sun," which halts its northward movement in the sky. At the precise moment of the equinox, the High Priest lays his hands on the stone and prays for more years of prosperity. You then give gratitude to the sun and its life-giving rays . . . [Record 10 seconds of silence here.]

At the end of the ritual, you touch your forehead to the Intihuatana stone. Spiritual energy flows through your body, your perception awakens to higher consciousness, your heart opens, and you are flooded with light. You can see visions of spiritual beings . . . [Record 20 seconds of silence here.]

Then you and your Inca guides enter the Temple of the Condor, where you sit in a circle around the condor-shaped stone, and you enjoy some time of deep self-reflection . . . [Record 20 seconds of silence here.]

The group treks to the Sacred Rock, where you gather for a sunset ritual of offerings of sweet fruits and flowers to Pachamama (Earth

Mother). After the ceremony, you touch your forehead to the Sacred Rock, where you pass through an inter-dimensional doorway to a higher realm. There you can see ancient divine beings of light and communicate with them. Then you sit on the ledge of the Sacred Rock for a final, deep silent meditation . . . [Record one minute of silence here.]

Now it is time to come forth from this visualization. Give gratitude to Spirit. Then pretend to vigorously blow out a candle as you come forth from the level of Spirit to your subconscious mind, which has been permanently transformed, lifted, and healed by this meditation. Then blow out another candle and affirm that your conscious mind is now one with the divine mind. Blow out a third candle and know that your body is now filled with robust health and energy. Then blow out a fourth candle as you return to this room and this place and time. Know that you are bringing all the blessings of Spirit into your environment.

Finally, blow out four more candles, come out of meditation, and then open your eyes . . . [Record 10 seconds of silence here.] With eyes wide open, now repeat the following affirmation:

> *I AM alert . . . I AM awake . . . I AM very alert . . . I AM very awake . . . I AM in control . . . I AM the only authority in my life . . . I AM divinely protected . . . by the light of my being . . . Thank you God, and SO IT IS.*

SWEAT LODGE JOURNEY

Please record this visualization on your device:

Please sit comfortably and close your eyes. Keep your eyes closed until I tell you to open them. Let us take a big deep breath of divine love. Breathe in . . . And out . . . Take a big deep breath of divine light. Breathe in . . . And out . . . And a big deep breath of relaxation. Breathe in . . . And out . . . Then breathe normally.

Visualize yourself at a Native American sweat lodge ceremony, a gentle place to pray according to your spiritual beliefs, cure illness, revitalize aching muscles, balance your energies, realize your true identity, contact your ancestral spirits, and connect with and honor the Creator. A sweat lodge provides a safe environment that feels like the warmth, peace, and security of Mother Earth's womb.

The small lodge is a domed circular shape, about eight feet in diameter and four feet high, formed with supple willow branches. A pit of about two feet in diameter and one foot deep has been dug in the center. Rugs and blankets cover the willow branches to enclose the lodge in complete blackout darkness. A curved branch serves as the door frame on the east side, which is closed by a flap. Rugs where people can sit circle the inside of the lodge.

A fire pit has been dug about thirty feet away from the sweat lodge, to the direct east of the doorway. The ancestral Spirits come from the sky and follow the path of smoke from the fire into the lodge. Cedar boughs are laid on this path, which blocks the participants from nearing the fire pit.

Large lava rocks known as the "Grandfathers," which absorb intense heat, are laid at the bottom of the fire pit. The fire keeper lights the fire several hours in advance of the ceremony. When twenty-eight Grandfathers are glowing red hot, it is time for the ceremony to begin. You are wearing comfortable, loose clothing, and you bring two towels, a bottle of water, and a drum to beat during the ceremony. Women wear long cotton dresses, and men wear shorts or sweatpants.

Before you enter the lodge, the leader smudges you with a feather by fanning you with smoke from burning sage. Women enter the lodge first and men follow. You circumambulate the exterior of the lodge clockwise, to honor the natural order and energies of the universe. Then you kneel in the doorway, bless the Grandfather Spirits, and enter the lodge on your hands and knees, keeping to the left, circling clockwise. After everyone is inside, woman are seated in the north side of the lodge and men in the south.

A large bucket of water is placed by the pit inside the lodge. The leader, who sits by the door, distributes cedar, sage, and sweet-grass for everyone to sprinkle onto the Grandfathers. The fire keeper brings in glowing hot rocks one-by-one on a pitchfork. You bless each hot stone with plant medicines as it is placed in the center shallow pit.

Immediately the sweet vapors rise. As you inhale its healing smoke, the sage blesses, cleanses, heals, and calms you. It washes off the outside world and centers you. The old, wise, powerful spirits of cedar protect you from negative influences. Inhaling its smoke exorcises unwanted spirits. As you inhale the sweet vanilla-like mist of sweet-grass, it blesses you with Mother Earth's breath and love. You imbibe this feminine essence as a reminder that earth provides all your needs.

Seven Grandfathers in the pit represent seven directions (west, north, east, south, up, down, and within). After all seven are placed, the fire keeper closes the flap and the ceremony begins. The lodge is pitch black inside, except for the glowing red Grandfathers in the center.

The leader beats a drum and calls forth spirit guides from the four compass directions. From the water bucket, she splashes one cup on the stones to represent each direction. As steam rises, the leader beats the drum and chants the following prayer:

Grandfather, Mysterious One,

We search for you along this Great Red Road you have set us on.

Sky Father, Tunkashila, We thank you for this world.

We thank you for our own existence.

We ask only for your blessing and for your instruction.

Grandfather, Sacred One,

Put our feet on the holy path that leads to you,

And give us the strength and the will

To lead ourselves and our children past the darkness we have entered.

Teach us to heal ourselves, to heal each other and to heal the world.

Let us begin this very day, this very hour, the Great Healing to come.

Let us walk the Red Road in Peace.

Mitakuye O'Yasin ["all my relations" in the Lakota language].

AHO [amen].

The sweat lodge ceremony consists of four rounds—one for each compass direction. The leader calls on the West while scattering plant medicines and splashing water on the Grandfathers. She says, "The first round is for recognition of the spirit world, which resides in the black West where the sun sets. In this round, you may ask our Creator for a 'spirit guide.' Sunsets give us glorious colors. Night can be scary, but darkness also means calming, healing sleep. May deep sleep and sweet dreams cleanse us from all evil. Renew and refresh us, O Lord."

When the leader's songs and prayers are finished, she hands a feather to the person on her left. That person honors, prays, and thanks the Grandfathers, and this subsequently continues until everyone shares. As each person prays, the leader splashes water onto the hot Grandfathers.

Now spend a few moments speaking audibly to honor, pray, and thank the Grandfathers, Grandmothers and the Creator for all that was, all that is, and all that will be . . . [Record 15 seconds of silence here.]

At the end of the first round, the leader yells "In the name of all my relations," and the fire keeper opens the flap. There is a ten-minute interlude for the guests to cool down. You may either exit the lodge and take a dip in a nearby clear mountain stream, or remain where you are. The leader then asks the fire keeper to bring in seven more glowing Grandfathers with a pitchfork, one at a time. When the leader says "door," the flap is closed again.

The second round begins. Each round is hotter than the previous, as the number of hot rocks increases by seven each time. The leader scatters medicine, splashes water on the Grandfathers, and says, "The second round calls upon the power of the white North for courage, endurance, strength, cleanliness, and honesty. North winds may bring stormy weather and snow. Let your warmth wrap us in a blanket of love to keep away all hurt and pain. May all our relations have warm houses and full tables against winter's chill, my Lord."

The leader then sings and beats a drum, and each participant prays for two-legged, four-legged, finned, and winged beings. Now take a few moments to speak audible prayers for these creatures . . . [Record 30 seconds of silence here.] At the end of this round, the flap opens, the fire keeper brings in seven more hot, glowing rocks, and the flap closes again.

As the third round begins, the leader scatters medicine, splashes water on the Grandfathers, and says, "The third round calls upon the direction of the daybreak star and rising sun. We pray for wisdom in all our endeavors as we follow the Red Road of the East. All good comes from the East. The freshening wind brings warm rain and sunshine. Please guide us to see you in everything we do, everyone we meet. Be kind in your blessings, oh Lord."

In this round, participants pray for specific people, places, things— for those suffering with addictions or heartache, or due to natural disasters, and for displaced animals in danger. Now spend time praying audibly for beings in pain . . . [Record one minute of silence here.] At the end of this round, the flap is opened and seven more hot, glowing rocks are brought in. Then the flap closes again.

As the fourth round begins, the leader scatters medicine, splashes water on the Grandfathers, and says, "The last round of the yellow South centers on spiritual growth and healing. The warming south winds bring new growth, gentle rain, and healing sunshine. Bless us with nourishing food and good things from the earth. Help us to know you as the giver of all gifts, oh Lord."

This round is for you to pray for yourself, for help with your weaknesses, trials and tribulations. Participants share deeply personal concerns and issues. Trust and confidentiality are paramount. Spend some time now praying audibly for yourself . . . [Record one minute of silence here.]

At the end of this round, the flap opens. All participants exit the lodge in a clockwise direction. When you get to the door, face the Grandfathers, give gratitude, and back out of the doorway from the lodge.

After exiting the lodge, take a refreshing dip in a beautiful, cool stream of fresh glacial water, which flows just a few yards from the lodge. As you give gratitude for this powerful experience, you feel renewed, refreshed, cleansed, and healed.

Now it is time to come forth from this visualization. Give gratitude to Spirit. Then pretend to vigorously blow out a candle as you come forth from the level of Spirit to your subconscious mind, which has been permanently transformed, lifted, and healed by this meditation. Then blow out another candle and affirm that your conscious mind is now one with the divine mind. Blow out a third candle and know that your body is now filled with robust health and energy. Then blow out a fourth candle as you return to this room and this place and time. Know that you are bringing all the blessings of Spirit into your environment.

Finally, blow out four more candles, come out of meditation, and then open your eyes . . . [Record 10 seconds of silence here.] With eyes wide open, now repeat the following affirmation:

> *I AM alert . . . I AM awake . . . I AM very alert . . . I AM very awake . . . I AM in control . . . I AM the only authority in my life . . . I AM divinely protected . . . by the light of my being . . . Thank you God, and SO IT IS.*

JOURNEY TO KUMBH MELA AT PRAYAG

Please record this visualization on your device:

Please sit comfortably and close your eyes. Keep your eyes closed until I tell you to open them. Let us take a big deep breath of divine love. Breathe in . . . And out . . . Take a big deep breath of divine light. Breathe in . . . And out . . . And a big deep breath of relaxation. Breathe in . . . And out . . . Then breathe normally.

Visualize yourself attending a vast, spectacular Hindu religious festival called "Maha Kumbh Mela" ("the great festival of the pot of immortal nectar"), visited by 100 million people over a six-week period. This festival occurs in Allahabad, India, at the confluence of three sacred rivers: the Ganges, Yamuna, and mythical Saraswati. In an elaborate tent city of about 12.5 square miles constructed on a sandbar, adepts and aspirants, saints and seekers, seers, sages, swamis, sannyasins, and ascetics assemble at the holiest of bathing spots in India.

In a most profound act of faith, tens of millions of pilgrims converge on Allahabad from every corner of India, many on foot, trudging hundreds of miles with huge bundles precariously balanced on their heads. Their footwear consists of rubber thong sandals or bare feet. Their journey begins months in advance. Devotees pile onto bullock and horse carts overstuffed with teaming humanity, or pack into rickety buses spewing black clouds of exhaust with crushes of arms, elbows, and toothy white grins hanging out the windows.

Imagine the crowd and commotion of pilgrims and religious leaders in every imaginable costume. Vibrant fuchsia, yellow, orange, electric blue, green, and violet saris blur past in a kaleidoscope of brilliant eye candy. Gurus are decked in cloths of spun gold, in saffron robes, in loincloths, or fully naked, covered in gray ash and garlanded with marigolds.

Bards of a hundred different traditions enchant pilgrims with legends as ancient as India herself. An elephant begs for coins with its trunk; robots and parrots tell fortunes. Fakirs recline on sharp spikes while yogis perform headstands. Sounds of conch shells trumpet and snake charmers' pipes rend the air. The mélange of priests, soldiers, religious mendicants, half-beggars, half-bandits, with a rare smattering of long-haired Europeans, exhibit an exotic, picturesque display, unique in the entire world.

As you wander among rows of giant, palatial tents, sponsored by religious organizations, topped with brightly colored flags and cloth towers, you sample a spiritual smorgasbord of countless sects. You visit some of the sages camped in thousands of small tents, where you share food and take a few puffs of hashish. You are blessed by the holy presence of these sadhus. A dreamlike, surrealistic quality imbues the entire scene.

At dawn the atmosphere is charged with the recitation of mantras and the deep meditation of countless adepts. As the sky brightens, pilgrims pour from every direction to bathe in the sacred waters. A smoky, balmy film can be perceived on the riverbanks from a distance. As you draw near, the fragrance of thousands of incense sticks and vapors of smoldering clarified butter from thousands of oil lamps waft along the riverbank. Religious chants echo all around, along with the trumpet of conch shells and clatter of brass bells. A spiritual extravaganza fills the air.

Ganga is said to be Mother Divine, who descended onto earth from her celestial home for the welfare of humanity. This eternal, nourishing river of life is the nerve center of India's ancient culture. Millions purify themselves through bathing rituals at the confluence, where the time-hallowed rivers are charged with spiritual vibrations by the meditations and prayers of thousands of saints since the dawn of time. During Kumbh Mela, the spiritual potency of the rivers increases manifold due to an auspicious planetary position that medicates the holy waters and transforms them into heavenly nectar.

On auspicious holy bathing dates, a colorful, magnificent, miles-long procession of religious ascetics from nineteen different sects begins before sunrise. As you witness the march of the ages in awe, holy saints pass by on sundry conveyances, showering flower petals, imparting blessings of divine grace, transmitting waves of powerful spiritual energy. Palpable spiritual vibrations pervade the atmosphere—pure enchantment for the soul.

Holy men and women approach the river in resplendence, mounted on magnificently outfitted horses, on tasseled, vermilion-coated, enormous chariots, marigold-embellished floats, or gold and silver palanquins hooded by magnificently embroidered umbrellas. Children attired as Hindu deities wear sparkling jewel-encrusted crowns and perch on superbly ornamented thrones. Clapping, chanting, shouting devotees follow, waving colorful flags and banners.

While the parade of saints march in regal splendor toward the holy waters, the sounds baffle description—the cries of ash-smeared sadhus mingle with neighing horses, blaring trumpets, beating drums, bleating conch shells, and chiming bells. In the midst of this cacophony, musicians and dancers perform, while devotees sing. The air is saturated with incense, flower fragrance, Vedic hymns, and sacred mantras.

As they approach the river at dawn, the glorious saints, many bearing elaborately carved silver staffs, relinquish their clothing and run with gusto and abandon toward the river to take their royal dip— shouting, singing, chanting and rejoicing. The first to hit the water in a tumult are legions of ferocious-looking Shiva devotees with naked ash-smeared bodies and long dreadlocks, often coiled atop their heads. These ascetics, who engage in austere practices and celibacy, consider themselves as guardians of the faith, as Mother India's spiritual army.

The naked saints rush to the river with the pomp and bravado of a charging army, brandishing giant silver swords, spears, flags, or tridents (the symbol of Lord Shiva). As they yell "Great Lord Hari," "All glory to Lord Shiva," and "All glory to Mother Ganga," they charge into the river to the trumpet of conch shells, first dipping their weapons into the water, then splashing and frolicking like children.

After sunrise, the sight at the river is amazing to behold. A sea of humanity stretches down a slope toward the beach, as far as the eye can see. The deep blue waters of the Yamuna mixing with the silver Ganges paints a highly emotionally-charged picture of great wonderment that touches your soul deeply and brings tears to your eyes.

After many of the holy sages bathe, you take your turn in the adjacent bathing area. Millions of bodies are crushing toward the spot where the rivers meet at the time of the auspicious planetary alignment. Getting to the river is easy. You are simply swept along in the tide with a sea of bodies, moving in two directions—either toward the river or away. After entering the river, pilgrims stand waist-deep, cupping the sacred water in their palms and offering it back to mother Ganges in reverence. Then they immerse themselves fully.

Once you enter the water, bathing at the holy confluence is a deeply moving, powerful experience of profound significance. This soul cleansing results in a heightened, keen sensory awareness, spiritual exaltation, gratitude, humility, and triumphant jubilation. You feel purified on every level: physically, mentally, emotionally, and spiritually. The spiritual merit gained by bathing during Kumbh Mela is equivalent to that obtained by fasting for a hundred years. As you wash away all limitations and overcome karmic consequences, the cycle of rebirth and death ends and your soul attains divine union—oneness with God.

After your holy dip, visualize yourself wandering amongst the throngs of devotees, like floating through a dream of dazzling transparent prisms. The radiant hues of celestial luminescence glow through every pilgrim, the vibrant multicolored saris, the radiant tents and brilliant flags flutter in the river breeze, and the ochre sand shimmers like a million tiny jewels.

There is nothing but the blissful glow of divine love everywhere, in each smile, the wrinkle on every face, the sparkle in each eye, the red powder or sandalwood paste smeared on every forehead. You float through the kaleidoscopic multitudes like a boat of vibrant serenity bobbing along an ocean of ecstasy. Nothing matters except this measureless place and this timeless moment . . . [Record 30 seconds of silence here.]

Now it is time to come forth from this visualization. Give gratitude to Spirit. Then pretend to vigorously blow out a candle as you come forth from the level of Spirit to your subconscious mind, which has been permanently transformed, lifted, and healed by this meditation. Then blow out another candle and affirm that your conscious mind is now one with the divine mind. Blow out a third candle and know that your body is now filled with robust health and energy. Then blow out a fourth candle as you return to this room and this place and time. Know that you are bringing all the blessings of Spirit into your environment.

Finally, blow out four more candles, come out of meditation, and then open your eyes . . . [Record 10 seconds of silence here.] With eyes wide open, now repeat the following affirmation:

I AM alert . . . I AM awake . . . I AM very alert . . . I AM very awake . . . I AM in control . . . I AM the only authority in my life . . . I AM divinely protected . . . by the light of my being . . . Thank you God, and SO IT IS.

End Notes

Introduction

1. *www.sacred-texts.com*

2. *biblehub.com*

Chapter 3

1. *www.ourcatholicprayers.com*

2. *www.myjewishlearning.com*

3. *www.beliefnet.com*

4. *www.buddhaweekly.com*

Chapter 6

1. *www.astrojyoti.com*

Chapter 9

1. *aumamen.com*

2. *www.templepurohit.com*

Chapter 10

1. *aumamen.com*

Chapter 11

1. *aumamen.com*

Chapter 12

1. *www.crystal-life.com*

2. *aumamen.com*

3. *aumamen.com*

Other Books by the Author

Divine Revelation. New York: Fireside/Touchstone/Simon & Schuster, 1996

Exploring Meditation. Newburyport, MA: New Page Books, 2002

Miracle Prayer. Berkeley, CA: Celestial Arts/Penguin Random House, 2006

Ascension. Newburyport, MA: New Page Books, 2010

Instant Healing. Newburyport, MA: New Page Books, 2013

The Power of Auras. Newburyport, MA: New Page Books, 2013

The Power of Chakras. Newburyport, MA: New Page Books, 2013

Awaken Your Divine Intuition. Newburyport, MA: New Page Books, 2016

Awaken Your Third Eye. Newburyport, MA: New Page Books, 2016

Color Your Chakras. Newburyport, MA: Red Wheel/Weiser, 2016

Maharishi & Me. New York: Skyhorse Publishing, 2018.

The Big Book of Chakras and Chakra Healing. Newburyport, MA: Weiser Books, 2019

Third Eye Meditations. Newburyport, MA: Weiser Books, 2020

How India Influenced the Beatles. Brentwood, TN: Posthill Press, 2021

Acknowledgments

I am grateful to those who have helped bring this book to press. Thank you to Jeff and Deborah Herman, who have been loyal friends and advisors for over twenty-five years. I thank Michael Pye and Laurie Kelly-Pye for your continued steadfast support. Thank you to Christine LeBlond, Kasandra Cook, Kathryn Sky-Peck and everyone else at Red Wheel/Weiser, who have worked diligently to bring this book to publication.

I give special thanks to my mentors, Maharishi Mahesh Yogi, Peter Victor Meyer, and all my inner teachers and divine beings of light, including the immortal Babaji. Their influence has been my unfaltering, steady, constant inspiration.

About the Author

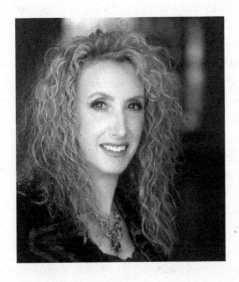

Dr. Susan Shumsky has dedicated her life to helping people take command of their lives in highly effective, powerful, positive ways. She is a leading spirituality expert, highly-acclaimed and greatly respected professional speaker, sought-after media guest, New Thought minister, and Doctor of Divinity.

Dr. Shumsky is a best-selling author of eighteen books, including *Divine Revelation, Ascension, Miracle Prayer, Exploring Meditation, Instant Healing, The Power of Auras, Awaken Your Third Eye, Awaken Your Divine Intuition, Color Your Chakras, The Big Book of Chakras and Chakra Healing, Third Eye Meditations,* and her memoir *Maharishi & Me.* Dr. Shumsky has won forty prestigious book awards. Many of her books were #1 Amazon.com bestsellers, and two were One Spirit

Book Club selections. Her books have been published in a total of thirty-six foreign editions.

Dr. Shumsky has practiced self-development disciplines since 1967. Dr. Shumsky practiced long hours of meditation in the Himalayas, Swiss Alps, and other secluded areas, under the personal guidance of enlightened master from India, Maharishi Mahesh Yogi, founder of Transcendental Meditation and guru of the Beatles, of Deepak Chopra, and other major celebrities. Dr. Shumsky served on Maharishi's personal staff for six years in Europe. She then studied New Thought and metaphysics and became a Doctor of Divinity.

Dr. Shumsky was not born with any supernormal faculties but developed her expertise through decades of patient daily study and practice. She has taught yoga, meditation, prayer, and intuition to thousands of students worldwide since 1970 as a pioneer in the consciousness field. She is founder of Divine Revelation®, a unique, field-proven technology for contacting the divine presence, hearing and testing the inner voice, and receiving clear divine guidance.

Dr. Shumsky travels extensively, producing and facilitating workshops, conferences, ocean cruise seminars, and tours to sacred destinations worldwide. She also offers teleseminars and private spiritual coaching, prayer therapy sessions, and spiritual break-through sessions. Over five decades of research into consciousness have contributed to her books, which can significantly reduce pitfalls in a seeker's quest for inner truth and shorten the pathway to Spirit.

On her websites, *www.drsusan.org* and *www.divinetravels.com*, you can:

- Join the mailing list.

- See Dr. Shumsky's itinerary.

- Read the first chapter of Dr. Shumsky's books.

- Enjoy Dr. Shumsky's free interviews, articles, and videos.

- Find Divine Revelation teachers in various areas.

- Order books, audio and video products, downloadable files, home study courses, and laminated affirmation cards.

- Order beautiful, full-color prints of Dr. Shumsky's illustrations.

- Register for telephone sessions and teleseminars with Dr. Shumsky.

- Register for a spiritual cruise, retreat, or tour.

When you join the mailing list at *www.drsusan.org,* you will receive a free, downloadable, guided mini-meditation plus access to Dr. Shumsky's free online community group forum and free weekly teleconference prayer circle.

As a gift for reading this book, please use the following special code to get a $100 discount on one of her spiritual cruises, retreats, or tours at *www.divinetravels.com:* MEDITATION108.

We want to hear from you. Please share your personal experiences of meditation or invite Dr. Shumsky to speak to your group: *divinerev@aol.com.* If you enjoyed this book, please write a customer review on Amazon, and please give this book to friends and family as gifts. You might also enjoy getting a copy of this book in an audio edition, so you can listen to and practice the guided meditations. It is available through Brilliance Audio.

To Our Readers

Weiser Books, an imprint of Red Wheel/Weiser, publishes books across the entire spectrum of occult, esoteric, speculative, and New Age subjects. Our mission is to publish quality books that will make a difference in people's lives without advocating any one particular path or field of study. We value the integrity, originality, and depth of knowledge of our authors.

Our readers are our most important resource, and we appreciate your input, suggestions, and ideas about what you would like to see published.

Visit our website at *www.redwheelweiser.com* to learn about our upcoming books and free downloads, and be sure to go to *www.redwheelweiser.com/newsletter* to sign up for newsletters and exclusive offers.

You can also contact us at *info@rwwbooks.com* or at

Red Wheel/Weiser, LLC
65 Parker Street, Suite 7
Newburyport, MA 01950